Student Workbook
to accompany the seventh edition of
Torres and Ehrlich Modern Dental Assisting

Student Workbook
TO ACCOMPANY

Torres and Ehrlich
Modern Dental Assisting

SEVENTH EDITION

Doni L. Bird, CDA, RDH, MA

Director, Dental Programs
Santa Rosa Junior College
Santa Rosa, California

Debbie S. Robinson, CDA, MS

Dental Assisting Educational Consultant,
formerly Coordinator, Dental Assisting Program
University of North Carolina
Hillsborough, North Carolina

SAUNDERS
An Imprint of Elsevier Science
Philadelphia London New York St. Louis Sydney Toronto

SAUNDERS
An Imprint of Elsevier Science

11830 Westline Industrial Drive
St. Louis, Missouri 63146

NOTICE

Dental Assisting is an ever-changing field. Standard safety precautions must be followed but as new research and clinical experience broaden our knowledge, changes in treatment and drug therapy may become necessary or appropriate. Readers are advised to check the most current product information provided by the manufacturer of each drug to be administered to verify the recommended dose, the method and duration of administration, and con-traindications. It is the responsibility of the treating physician, relying on experience and knowledge of the patient, to determine dosages and the best treatment for each individual patient. Neither the Publisher nor the author assumes any liability for any injury and/or damage to persons or property arising from this publication.

The Publisher

Previous edition copyrighted 1999.

International Standard Book Number 0-7216-9770-4

Acquisitions Editor: Shirley Kuhn
Developmental Editor: Helaine Tobin
Publishing Services Manager: Gayle May
Project Manager: Carla Babrick
Design Coordinator: Julia Dummitt

KI/MVB
Printed in the United States of America

Last digit is the print number: 9   8   7   6   5   4   3   2   1

Table of Contents

Introduction

TO THE STUDENT

The student workbook is designed to help you prepare for and master the preclinical, clinical, and administrative procedures presented in *Torres and Ehrlich Modern Dental Assisting,* Seventh Edition. The workbook includes the following.

CHAPTER EXERCISES

Each chapter includes (1) short answer questions, which are taken from the chapter's learning outcomes; (2) fill in the blank questions, which stem from the key terms of the chapter; (3) multiple choice questions that parallel the recall questions; and (4) case studies that tie in the chapter plus introducing knowledge from additional chapters. These types of questions are intended to help you study, interact with, and better understand the information presented in the corresponding chapter of the textbook. Please take the time to work through them carefully.

COMPETENCY SHEETS

A competency is a system that is used to evaluate the dental assistant's mastery of preclinical, clinical, administrative, and advanced skills. The competency forms are designed to give you the opportunity to practice a skill until you have mastered it. A space on the form allows for at least three different evaluations. The first time you may wish to evaluate your own performance. The second time you might ask a classmate to give you feedback. When you feel comfortable with that skill, the evaluator would be your instructor, clinic supervisor, or dentist.

The ability to objectively evaluate your performance is an important skill to develop. Once you are working in a dental practice, many of the important tasks assigned to you are performed without direct supervision. In this situation you are responsible for maintaining your skills and the quality of your work.

FLASHCARDS

The study cards contain specific information from sections within the textbook to help you prepare for courses and for the certification examination. The information on these cards is organized so that they can be removed from the text for use as an easy study tool. The sections covered are the sciences, medical emergencies, infection control, radiography, dental materials, instruments, and dental procedures.

The authors of *Torres and Ehrlich Modern Dental Assisting,* Seventh Edition, wish you success in your studies and your chosen profession of dental assisting.

1 | History of Dentistry

SHORT ANSWER QUESTIONS

1. Describe the role of Hippocrates in history.
2. State the basic premise of the Hippocratic Oath.
3. Name the first woman to graduate from a college of dentistry.
4. Name the first woman to practice dentistry in the United States.
5. List the contributions of Horace H. Hayden and Chapin A. Harris to dentistry.
6. Describe two major contributions of Dr. G.V. Black.
7. Name the first dentist to employ a dental assistant.
8. Name the person who discovered x-rays.
9. Name the person who first used nitrous oxide for extractions.

FILL IN THE BLANK

Select the best term from the list below and complete the following statements.

Commission on Dental Accreditation of the American Dental Association
Dental treatise
Forensic dentist
Periodontal disease
Preceptorship

1. A _____ is a formal article or book based on evidence and facts.

2. To study under the guidance of one already in the profession is a _____ .

3. A _____ establishes the identity of a person based on dental records only.

4. _____ is a disease of the structures that support the teeth (gums and bone).

5. The _____ accredits dental, dental assisting, dental hygiene, and dental laboratory educational programs.

MULTIPLE CHOICE

Complete each question by circling the best answer.

1. Hesi-Re was:

   a. the first female dentist.
   b. the earliest recorded dentist.
   c. the first dental assistant.
   d. the first dental hygienist.

2. How long has there been dental disease?

   a. Since the nineteenth century
   b. Since the eighteenth century
   c. Since humankind began
   d. Since the stone age

3. Who is known as the Father of Medicine?

   a. Hippocrates
   b. G.V. Black
   c. Pierre Fauchard
   d. Paul Revere

4. What does the Hippocratic Oath promise?

   a. To heal all
   b. To treat dental problems of all ages
   c. To do no harm
   d. To include dentistry in medicine

5. What type of dentistry did the Romans provide?

   a. Oral hygiene
   b. Gold crowns
   c. Tooth extraction
   d. All of the above

6. Which artist first distinguished molars and premolars?

   a. Monet
   b. Leonardo da Vinci
   c. van Gogh
   d. Peter Max

7. Who is referred to as the Father of Modern Surgery?

   a. Ambroise Paré
   b. Hippocrates
   c. G.V. Black
   d. Pierre Fauchard

8. Who is referred to as the Father of Modern Dentistry?

    a. Ambroise Paré
    b. Hippocrates
    c. G.V. Black
    d. Pierre Fauchard

9. Who was John Baker's famous patient?

    a. Paul Revere
    b. George Washington
    c. Leonardo da Vinci
    d. Hippocrates

10. What famous colonial patriot first used forensic evidence?

    a. Paul Revere
    b. George Washington
    c. Abraham Lincoln
    d. Betsy Ross

11. Who was one of the first dentists to travel throughout the colonies?

    a. Paul Revere
    b. George Washington
    c. Abraham Lincoln
    d. Robert Woffendale

12. Who is credited with founding the first dental school in the United States?

    a. Chapin Harris
    b. Horace Wells
    c. G.V. Black
    d. Edmund Kells

13. Who earned the title of Grand Old Man of Dentistry?

    a. Chapin Harris
    b. Horace Wells
    c. G.V. Black
    d. Edmund Kells

14. Who is credited with employing the first dental assistant?

    a. Chapin Harris
    b. Horace Wells
    c. G.V. Black
    d. Edmund Kells

15. Who was the first dentist to use nitrous oxide in dentistry?

    a. Chapin Harris
    b. Horace Wells
    c. G.V. Black
    d. Edmund Kells

16. Who was the first woman dentist in America?

    a. Emiline Roberts-Jones
    b. Lucy Beaman Hobbs
    c. G.V. Black
    d. W.B. Saunders

17. Who was the first woman in the world to graduate from dental school?

    a. Emiline Roberts-Jones
    b. Lucy Beaman Hobbs
    c. G.V. Black
    d. W.B. Saunders

ACTIVITY

Every person has his or her own unique genetic makeup. A lot of your features, size, and shape are because of your inherited genes. Go to family members, especially older generations, and explore specific inherited oral and facial anomalies that make you unique. Specific questions to ask are the following:

1. Do members of your family keep their natural teeth for a long time or do many have dentures or partials?
2. Was the size and shape of anyone's jaws unique?
3. Did anyone have a unique type of bite?
4. Was the shape of anyone's teeth unique?
5. Did any past relatives adopt different types of dental care or treatment that worked for them?

2 | The Professional Dental Assistant

SHORT ANSWER QUESTIONS

1. Discuss the concept of professionalism.
2. Describe the characteristics of a professional dental assistant.
3. Describe the personal qualities of a dental assistant.
4. Describe the role and purpose of the American Dental Assistants Association.
5. Describe the benefits of membership in the American Dental Assisting Association.
6. Describe the role of the Dental Assisting National Board.

FILL IN THE BLANK

Select the best term from the list below and complete the following statements.

American Dental Assistants Association
Certified Dental Assistant
Dental Assisting National Board
Professional

1. A(n) _____ is one who meets the high standards of the profession.

2. _____ is the professional organization that represents the profession of dental assisting.

3. The national agency that is responsible for administering the certification examination and issuing certification is the _____.

4. A(n) _____ is the credential of someone who has passed the certification examination and remains current through continuing education.

MULTIPLE CHOICE

Complete each question by circling the best answer.

1. The essentials of professional appearance are:

   a. good health.
   b. good grooming.
   c. appropriate dress.
   d. all of the above.

2. How does one demonstrate responsibility?

   a. Arriving on time
   b. Volunteering to help
   c. Showing initiative
   d. All of the above

3. What is the purpose of the ADAA?

   a. To advance the careers of dental assistants
   b. To promote the dental assisting profession
   c. To enhance the delivery of quality dental health care
   d. All of the above

4. What credential is issued by DANB?

   a. Registered dental assistant
   b. Certified dental assistant
   c. Licensed dental assistant
   d. Bachelor's degree

ACTIVITY

Develop your own questions about the profession of dental assisting. Visit your own dentist and discuss these questions with the dentist and dental assistant.

3 Roles of the Dental Health Care Team

SHORT ANSWER QUESTIONS

1. Name the members of the dental health team, and explain their roles in a dental practice.
2. Identify the minimal educational requirements for each member of the dental health care team.
3. Describe the supportive services provided by non–team members.
4. Identify the founder of the first dental hygiene school.
5. Name and describe each of the recognized dental specialties.

FILL IN THE BLANK

Select the best term from the list below and complete the following statements.

Dental assistant
Dental hygienist
Dental laboratory technician
Dental public health
Dentist
Endodontist
Oral and maxillofacial radiology
Oral and maxillofacial surgery
Oral pathology
Orthodontics
Pediatric dentistry
Periodontics
Prosthodontics

1. A person who is trained to provide support to a dentist is a(n) _____.

2. The specialty concerned with the diagnosis and treatment of the supporting structures is _____.

3. The specialty concerned with the diagnosis of disease through various forms of imaging including x-rays is _____.

4. A(n) _____ is a legally qualified practitioner of dentistry.

5. Someone who performs technical services specified by a written prescription from a dentist is a(n) _____.

6. A(n) _____ is a licensed auxiliary who provides preventive, therapeutic, and educational services.

7. The specialty of promoting dental health through organized community efforts is _____.

8. _____ is the specialty concerned with diseases of the oral structures.

9. A(n) _____ is a dentist that specializes in diseases of the pulp.

10. _____ is the specialty of surgery of the head and neck.

11. _____ is the specialty concerned with the correction of malocclusions.

12. _____ is the specialty concerned with restoration and replacement of natural teeth.

13. _____ is the area of dentistry specializing in children from birth to adolescence.

MULTIPLE CHOICE

Complete each question by circling the best answer.

1. Who would *not* be considered a member of the dental health care team?
   a. Dental hygienist
   b. Dental supply person
   c. Dental laboratory technician
   d. Dental assistant

2. What is the minimal length of education for dental hygiene licensure?

   a. 1 year
   b. 2 years
   c. 3 years
   d. 4 years

3. What is the minimal length for an ADA-accredited dental assisting program?

   a. 1 year
   b. 2 years
   c. 3 years
   d. 4 years

4. What is the minimal length for an ADA-accredited dental laboratory technician program?

   a. 1 year
   b. 2 years
   c. 3 years
   d. 4 years

5. What is the minimal length for an ADA-accredited dental program?

   a. 1 year
   b. 2 years
   c. 3 years
   d. 4 years

6. What must dental laboratory technicians have in hand before they can perform and deliver an indirect restoration or prosthesis?

   a. The patient record
   b. Letter from the dentist
   c. Prescription
   d. Drawing of the indirect restoration or prosthesis

CASE STUDY

You have just completed your education and training in an accredited dental assisting program. You are scheduled to take the dental assisting national board in a month. During this time, you plan to send out your resume and interview. You expect to find a clinical position quickly.

1. Can you start a position before taking the national boards?
2. How will working in a dental office before taking national boards help prepare you for the exam?
3. Is there any way that working in a dental office before taking the national boards would hinder you in preparing for the exam?
4. If you can work in a dental office without being certified, why bother taking the national boards?
5. What happens to someone who takes the national boards and does not pass a section on the exam?

4 | Dental Ethics

SHORT ANSWER QUESTIONS

1. Explain the basic principles of ethics.
2. Discuss the Code of Ethics of the American Dental Assistants Association.
3. Explain the difference between being legal and being ethical.
4. Identify sources of early learning of ethics.
5. Describe the model for ethical decision making.
6. Give personal examples of ethical and unethical behaviors.

FILL IN THE BLANK

Select the best term from the list below and complete the following statements.

Autonomy
Code of ethics
Ethics
Laws

1. _____ are minimal standards of behavior established by statutes.

2. Voluntary standards of behavior established by a profession are the _____.

3. _____ is standing up for one's self and beliefs.

4. _____ are morals, standards of conduct, and character.

MULTIPLE CHOICE

Complete each question by circling the best answer.

1. The basic principles of ethics include:

    a. autonomy.
    b. justice.
    c. do no harm.
    d. all of the above

2. What is established as a guide to professional behavior?

    a. Code of conduct
    b. Code of ethics
    c. Code of honor
    d. Code of medicine

3. Laws are established and influenced by:

    a. legislatures.
    b. individual interpretation.
    c. court decisions.
    d. a and c

4. Ethics consists of:

    a. statutes.
    b. individual interpretation.
    c. court decisions.
    d. a and c

ACTIVITIES

Aside from the examples in your textbook, provide an example of each of the following ethical principles and ways that they could relate to a situation within your dental assisting class.

1. Justice
2. Autonomy
3. Well-being
4. Doing no harm

If you were asked to write a code of ethics for your dental assisting class, what would be some of the issues to include? Why would this be an important document to follow?

5 | Dentistry and the Law

SHORT ANSWER QUESTIONS

1. Discuss the purpose of a state dental practice act.
2. Explain the purpose of licensing dental health professionals.
3. Describe the types of dental auxiliary supervision.
4. Explain the two categories of law.
5. Describe ways to prevent malpractice suits.
6. Demonstrate how to make corrections on a patient's record.
7. Give an example of respondeat superior.
8. Explain the difference between implied consent and written consent.
9. Give an example of res gestae.
10. Discuss the indications of child abuse and neglect.
11. Define the term *mandated reporter*.

FILL IN THE BLANK

Select the best term from the list below and complete the following statements.

Abandonment
Board of dentistry
Civil law
Contract law
Criminal law
Dental auxiliary
Direct supervision
Due care
Expanded functions
Expressed contract
General supervision
Implied consent
Implied contract
Licensure
Malpractice
Mandated reporters
Patient of record
Reciprocity
Res gestae
Respondeat superior
State dental practice act
Written consent

1. A(n) _____ can be a dental assistant, dental hygienist, or dental laboratory technician.

2. A(n) _____ is an individual who has been examined and diagnosed by the dentist and has had treatment planned.

3. A(n) _____ is an agreement for services in exchange for payment.

4. _____ is a level of supervision in which the dentist is physically present at the time the expanded functions are being performed by the dental auxiliary.

5. A(n) _____ is a specific intraoral function delegated to an auxiliary that requires increased skill and training.

6. _____ is a legal doctrine that holds the employer liable for the acts of the employee.

7. _____ specifies the legal requirements for an individual to practice dentistry in the state.

8. _____ is an agency that adopts rules and regulations and implements the state dental practice act.

9. A(n) _____ gives a person the legal right to practice in a specific state.

10. _____ is a system that allows individuals in one state to obtain a license in another state without retesting.

11. Terminating the dentist-patient relationship without reasonable notice to the patient is _____.

12. _____ is just, proper, and sufficient care, or the absence of negligence.

13. A(n) _____ is a violation against the state or government.

14. _____ is a level of supervision in which the dentist has given instructions, but need not be physically present at the time the expanded functions are being performed by the dental auxiliary.

15. _____ is professional negligence.

16. _____ is the patient's action indicating consent for treatment.

17. A(n) _____ deals with the relations of individuals, with corporations, or with other organizations.

18. A(n) _____ is a type of contract that may be either verbal or written.

19. A contract that is established by actions and not words is a(n) _____.

20. A(n) _____ is a written explanation of the diagnostic findings, the prescribed treatment, and the reasonable expectations as to the results of treatment.

21. _____ concerns a statement made by anyone at the time of an alleged negligent act. Under this concept, such a statement is admissible as evidence in a court of law.

22. A(n) _____ is a professional who is required by state law to report known or suspected child abuse.

MULTIPLE CHOICE

Complete each question by circling the best answer.

1. The purpose of being licensed is to:
   a. make more money.
   b. protect the public from incompetent practitioners.
   c. keep count of the number of professionals in the field.
   d. have laws to follow.

2. Who interprets the state dental practice act?
   a. Governor of the state
   b. American Dental Association
   c. State legislature
   d. Administrative board of dentistry

3. Reciprocity allows a licensed practitioner to:
   a. treat patients from another practice.
   b. prescribe drugs.
   c. practice in another state.
   d. specialize in a field of dentistry.

4. Respondeat superior states that a(n):
   a. patient can be seen by another dentist without records.
   b. employer is responsible for the actions of his or her employees.
   c. dentist can treat patients in another state.
   d. dentist can specialize and practice that specialty.

5. If a dentist is physically present when a dental auxiliary is performing an expanded function, the dentist is providing:
   a. direct supervision.
   b. physical supervision.
   c. general supervision.
   d. legal supervision.

6. When a dentist discontinues treatment after it has begun, he or she has performed:
   a. a felony.
   b. abuse.
   c. abandonment.
   d. a disservice.

7. When may a dentist refuse to treat a patient?
   a. Diagnosed with cancer
   b. Never
   c. Diagnosed with HIV
   d. If the dentist feels a patient would be better off if referred

8. When patients receive proper, sufficient care, they are receiving:

   a. poor care.
   b. due care.
   c. professional care.
   d. dental care.

9. A category of law is:

   a. civil.
   b. professional.
   c. contract.
   d. a and c

10. What are the two types of contracts?

    a. Professional
    b. Expressed
    c. Implied
    d. b and c

11. How can professionals best defend themselves from malpractice suits?

    a. Have a patient sign a form
    b. Prevention and communication
    c. Have their lawyer meet with the patient
    d. Scheduling and documenting

12. What is necessary for a successful malpractice suit?

    a. Duty
    b. Derelict
    c. Direct
    d. All of the above

13. A statement made by anyone at the time of an alleged negligent act is admissible as evidence in a court of law under the concept of:

    a. communication.
    b. res gestae.
    c. pro bono.
    d. due care.

14. Actions demonstrate:

    a. implied consent.
    b. verbal consent.
    c. written consent.
    d. legal consent.

15. Where should a broken appointment be recorded?

    a. Daily schedule
    b. Ledger
    c. Patient record
    d. Recall list

16. What is the purpose of reporting suspected cases of child abuse?

    a. To start the legal proceedings
    b. To have documentation
    c. To protect the child from further abuse
    d. To justify your innocence

17. Who are mandated reporters?

    a. Professionals required by state law to report known or suspected cases of child abuse
    b. Reporters from a newspaper following a story
    c. People elected to give their advice
    d. Written document on known or suspected cases of child abuse

ACTIVITY

Obtain a copy of your dental society newsletter, and review the topics that are being discussed within your state. Refer to the section covering suspensions and revocations of licenses. Discuss the situations and describe your position.

6 | General Anatomy

SHORT ANSWER QUESTIONS

1. Define each of the key terms in this chapter.
2. Explain the difference between anatomy and physiology.
3. Identify the imaginary planes used to divide the body into sections.
4. Identify the four levels of organization in the human body.
5. Describe the components of a cell.
6. Name the four types of tissues in the human body.
7. Name the two major body cavities.
8. Name the regions of the body.

FILL IN THE BLANK

Select the best term from the list below and complete the following statements.

Anatomical position
Anatomy
Anterior
Appendicular
Axial
Cranial cavity
Cytoplasm
Distal
Epithelial
Horizontal plane
Medial
Midsagittal
Nucleus
Organelles
Parietal
Physiology
Proximal
Sagittal plane
Superficial
Superior
Visceral

1. _____ is the study of the shape and structure of the human body.

2. _____ is the study of the functions of the human body.

3. The body is _____ when it is erect and facing forward with the arms at the sides and the palms facing up.

4. _____ is any vertical plane that divides the body from top to bottom, into left and right sections.

5. _____ is a vertical plane that divides the body into equal left and right halves.

6. _____ is dividing the body into superior (upper) and inferior (lower) portions.

7. The gel like fluid inside the cell is

    _____.

8. A(n) _____ is a specialized part of the cell that performs a definite function.

9. The center of a cell is the

    _____.

10. The _____ is a cavity that houses the brain.

11. _____ is a type of tissue that forms the covering for all body surfaces.

12. _____ is a part that is above another portion, or closer to the head.

13. _____ means toward the front surface.

14. _____ means toward, or nearer to the midline of the body.

15. _____ means that the part is closer to the trunk of the body.

16. _____ is the opposite of proximal: the part that is farther away from the trunk of the body.

17. _____ is the part that is located on or near the surface.

18. _____ pertains to internal organs or the covering of organs.

19. The wall of a body cavity is the

_____.

20. The region of the body that consists of the head, neck, and trunk is the _____.

21. The region of the body that consists of the limbs is the _____.

MULTIPLE CHOICE

Complete each question by circling the best answer.

1. Anatomy is the study of:

   a. function.
   b. form and structure.
   c. internal organs.
   d. veins and arteries.

2. Physiology is the study of:

   a. function.
   b. form and structure.
   c. internal organs.
   d. veins and arteries.

3. What imaginary line divides the body into upper and lower portions?

   a. Frontal
   b. Midsagittal
   c. Horizontal
   d. Sagittal

4. What imaginary line divides the body into equal right and left halves?

   a. Frontal
   b. Midsagittal
   c. Horizontal
   d. Sagittal

5. Name the portion of the cell that carries the genetic information.

   a. Cytoplasm
   b. Cell wall
   c. Mitochondria
   d. Nucleus

6. Body tissue that binds and supports other tissues is:

   a. epithelial.
   b. muscle.
   c. connective.
   d. nerve.

7. The organization levels of the body are cells, tissues, organs, and:

   a. bones.
   b. systems.
   c. brain.
   d. reproductive.

8. The two major cavities in the body are:

   a. sagittal and ventral.
   b. dorsal and median.
   c. cranial and thoracic.
   d. dorsal and ventral.

9. The axial portion of the body consists of:

   a. head.
   b. neck.
   c. trunk.
   d. all of the above

10. The appendicular portion of the body consists of:

    a. head.
    b. arms.
    c. legs.
    d. b and c

ACTIVITY

There are four types of tissue in the human body.

1. Describe each type of tissue.
2. Which tissues affect the oral facial part of the body?
3. Are there any types of tissue that may affect oral health? If yes, how and why?

7 | General Physiology

SHORT ANSWER QUESTIONS

1. Name and locate each of the body systems.
2. Explain the purpose of each body system.
3. Describe the components of each system.
4. Explain how each system functions.
5. Describe the signs and symptoms of common disorders related to each human body system.

FILL IN THE BLANK

Select the best term from the list below and complete the following statements.

Appendicular
Arteries
Articulations
Axial skeleton
Cancellous bone
Cartilage
Central nervous system
Compact bone
Integumentary system
Involuntary muscles
Joints
Muscle insertion
Muscle origin
Neurons
Osteoblasts
Pericardium
Periosteum
Peripheral nervous system
Peristalsis
Sharpey's fibers
Veins

1. The portion of the skeleton that consists of the skull, spinal column, ribs, and sternum is the _____.

2. _____ is the portion of the skeleton that consists of the upper extremities and shoulder girdle plus the lower extremities and pelvic girdle.

3. A specialized connective tissue that covers all bones of the body is the _____.

4. Cells that are associated with bone formation are _____.

5. The _____ anchors the periosteum to the bone.

6. _____ forms the outer layer of the bones, where it is needed for strength.

7. The lighter bone that is found in the interior of bones is the

_____.

8. _____ is a tough connective nonvascular elastic tissue.

9. Areas where two or more bones come together are _____.

10. _____ is another term for joints.

11. _____ are muscles that function automatically, without conscious control.

12. The location where a muscle begins is the

_____.

13. The location where a muscle ends is the

_____.

14. The _____ is a double-walled sac that encloses the heart.

15. _____ are large blood vessels that carry blood away from the heart.

16. Blood vessels that carry blood to the heart are _____.

17. The _____ is composed of the brain and spinal cord.

18. The _____ is composed of the cranial nerves and the spinal nerves.

19. _____ are direct nerve impulses.

20. A rhythmic action that moves food through the digestive tract is

_____.

21. The _____ involves the skin.

MULTIPLE CHOICE

Complete each question by circling the best answer.

1. The skeleton is divided into the axial and the:
   a. peripheral.
   b. appendicular.
   c. frontal.
   d. parietal.

2. Name the connective tissue that covers all bones.
   a. Nervous
   b. Muscle
   c. Epithelial
   d. Periosteum

3. The two types of bone are compact and:
   a. cortical.
   b. trabeculae.
   c. cancellous.
   d. periosteum.

4. Cartilage is found:
   a. at the end of bones.
   b. where bones join together.
   c. inside of bones.
   d. in the tissue.

5. *Articulation* is another term for:
   a. cartilage.
   b. bone.
   c. bone marrow.
   d. joint.

6. The type(s) of muscle tissue are:
   a. smooth.
   b. striated.
   c. cardiac.
   d. all of the above

7. The muscle that appears striated but resembles smooth muscle in its action is:
   a. smooth.
   b. striated.
   c. cardiac.
   d. skeletal.

8. A common muscular disorder is:
   a. muscular dystrophy.
   b. endocarditis.
   c. multiple sclerosis.
   d. gout.

9. A function of the circulatory system is to:
   a. provide fluids.
   b. provide the body with nutrients.
   c. regulate body temperature and chemical stability.
   d. destroy microorganisms.

10. The heart chambers consist of the atria and:
    a. pulmonic.
    b. aortic.
    c. mitral.
    d. ventricles.

11. A function of a blood vessel is to:
    a. carry blood away from the heart.
    b. connect the arterial and venous system.
    c. carry blood toward the heart.
    d. all of the above

12. The primary function of the lymph system is to:
    a. carry blood away from the heart.
    b. provide the body with nutrients.
    c. regulate body temperature and chemical stability.
    d. destroy harmful microorganisms.

13. What tissue(s) make up the lymph system?
    a. Lymph vessels
    b. Lymph nodes
    c. Lymph fluid
    d. All of the above

14. What systems make up the nervous system?

    a. Central nervous system
    b. Autonomic nervous system
    c. Peripheral nervous system
    d. a and c

15. The autonomic nervous system is divided into the parasympathetic and:

    a. sympathetic.
    b. autonomic.
    c. peripheral.
    d. central.

16. The type of neurons that carry impulses toward the brain and spinal cord are the:

    a. associative.
    b. motor.
    c. sensory.
    d. synapse.

17. The main function of the respiratory system is to:

    a. carry blood throughout the body.
    b. deliver oxygen to the body.
    c. give the body the ability to move.
    d. contribute to the immune system.

18. The role of the digestive system is to:

    a. provide nutrition for the body.
    b. deliver oxygen to the body.
    c. give the body the ability to move.
    d. contribute to the immune system.

19. Which would not be an action of the digestive system?

    a. Ingestion
    b. Sensory
    c. Movement
    d. Absorption

20. The primary function of the endocrine system is to:

    a. control growth.
    b. maintain homeostasis.
    c. form and eliminate urine.
    d. a and b

21. The primary function of the urinary system is:

    a. transport of oxygen to cells.
    b. defense against disease.
    c. formation and elimination of urine.
    d. regulation of body temperature.

22. The skin falls under which system?

    a. Skeletal
    b. Integumentary
    c. Nervous
    d. Muscular

23. An example of an appendage is the:

    a. hair.
    b. nails.
    c. glands.
    d. all of the above

CASE STUDY

A resting heart beats approximately 70 beats per minute. Take a rubber ball and hold it in the palm of your dominant hand. Straighten your arm out to the side. Squeeze the ball again and again for 1 minute and record your count.

1. How many times did you squeeze the ball in one minute?
2. Was this faster or slower than a normal heart beat for 1 minute?
3. What could you do when the muscles of your arm got tired?
4. Explain why cardiac muscle in your heart cannot do the same.

8 | Oral Embryology and Oral Histology

SHORT ANSWER QUESTIONS

1. Define embryology and histology.
2. Describe the three periods of prenatal development.
3. Explain types of prenatal influences on dental development.
4. Describe the function of osteoclasts and osteoblasts.
5. Explain the difference between the clinical and anatomical crown.
6. Name and describe the tissues of the teeth.
7. Name and describe the three types of dentin.
8. Describe the structure and location of the dental pulp.
9. Name and describe the components of the periodontium.
10. Describe the functions of the periodontal ligaments.
11. Describe the types of oral mucosa and give an example of each.

FILL IN THE BLANK

Select the best term from the list below and complete the following statements.

Ameloblasts
Cementoblasts
Cementoclasts
Conception
Embryology
Embryonic period
Exfoliation
Histology
Masticatory mucosa
Meiosis
Odontoblasts
Osteoclasts
Periodontium
Prenatal development
Stratified squamous epithelium
Succedaneous

1. _____ is the study of prenatal development.

2. _____ is the study of the structure and function of the tissues on a microscopic level.

3. _____ begins at the start of pregnancy and continues to birth.

4. Reproductive cell production that ensures the correct number of chromosomes is

_____

5. The _____ period extends from the beginning of the second week to the end of the eighth week.

6. The union of the male sperm and the ovum of the female is

_____.

7. _____ teeth are permanent teeth with primary predecessors; they include the anterior teeth and premolars.

8. The tissues that support the teeth in the alveolar bone are the

_____.

9. Enamel-forming cells are

_____.

10. _____ are dentin-forming cells.

11. _____ are cells that form cementum.

12. Cells that resorb cementum are

_____.

13. _____ are cells that resorb bone.

14. The normal process of shedding primary teeth is _____.

15. Oral mucosa is made up of

    _____.

16. Oral mucosa that covers the hard palate, dorsum of the tongue, and gingiva is

    _____.

MULTIPLE CHOICE

Complete each question by circling the best answer.

1. Name the first period of prenatal development.

   a. Embryonic period
   b. Fetal period
   c. Preimplantation period
   d. Embryo

2. Which period of prenatal development is the most critical?

   a. Embryonic period
   b. Fetal period
   c. Preimplantation period
   d. Embryo

3. The embryonic layer which differentiates into cartilage, bones, and muscles is:

   a. endoderm.
   b. ectoderm.
   c. mesoderm.
   d. pHisoDerm.

4. Which branchial arch forms the bones, muscles, nerves of the face, and the lower lip?

   a. First
   b. Second
   c. Third
   d. Fourth

5. Which branchial arch forms the side and front of the neck?

   a. First
   b. Second
   c. Third
   d. Fourth

6. The primary palate is formed by the union of the medial and lateral:

   a. maxillary processes.
   b. premaxilla.
   c. nasal processes.
   d. palatine processes.

7. When does the development of the human face occur?

   a. Second and third week
   b. Third and fourth week
   c. Fifth and eighth week
   d. Ninth and twelfth week

8. At birth, how many teeth are in various stages of development?

   a. 20
   b. 32
   c. 44
   d. 52

9. What factor can have a prenatal influence on dental development?

   a. Genetics
   b. Environment
   c. Physical
   d. a and b

10. Name the process for the laying down or adding of bone.

    a. Deposition
    b. Discharge
    c. Resorption
    d. Drift

11. Name the process of bone loss or removal.

    a. Deposition
    b. Discharge
    c. Resorption
    d. Drift

12. The three primary periods in tooth formation are growth, calcification, and:

    a. bud.
    b. eruption.
    c. cap.
    d. bell.

13. The final stage in the growth period is the:

    a. bud.
    b. cap.
    c. bell.
    d. calcification.

14. What is formed in the occlusal surface when multiple cusps join together?

    a. Dentinoenamel junction
    b. Fissure
    c. Pit
    d. b and c

15. What is the name of the process when teeth move into a functional position in the oral cavity?

    a. Eruption
    b. Exfoliation
    c. Development
    d. Resorption

16. The portion of a tooth that is visible in the mouth is the:

    a. anatomical crown.
    b. enamel crown.
    c. facial crown.
    d. clinical crown.

17. The cementoenamel junction is located:

    a. on the occlusal surface.
    b. between the dentin and enamel.
    c. between the pulp and cementum.
    d. between the cementum and enamel.

18. The hardest substance in the human body is:

    a. bone.
    b. enamel.
    c. dentin.
    d. cartilage.

19. What is the name of the largest mineral component in enamel?

    a. Calcium
    b. Magnesium
    c. Iron
    d. Palladium

20. Pain is transmitted through dentin by way of:

    a. dentinal tubules.
    b. dentinal fibers.
    c. odontoblasts.
    d. nerves.

21. The type of dentin that is also known as reparative dentin is:

    a. primary dentin.
    b. secondary dentin.
    c. tertiary dentin.
    d. odontoblasts.

22. The pulp is made up of:

    a. blood vessels.
    b. bone.
    c. nerves.
    d. a and c

23. What type of cells forms the intercellular substance of the pulp?

    a. Odontoblasts
    b. Fibroblasts
    c. Cementoblasts
    d. Dentinoblasts

24. The primary function of the periodontal ligament is to:

    a. support the tooth.
    b. maintain the tooth.
    c. retain the tooth.
    d. all of the above

25. Which type of oral mucosa forms the inside of the cheeks, lips, and soft palate?

    a. Masticatory mucosa
    b. Specialized mucosa
    c. Lining mucosa
    d. Gingival mucosa

CASE STUDY

Make a chart with each of the traits listed below. Survey 10 people (friends, family members, and similar) for the presence of these traits:

1. Freckles
2. Dimples
3. Cleft or smooth chin
4. Missing teeth
5. Crowded teeth

Compare the number of people who have one form of a trait with those who have more than one trait. Compare your charts to see if there is any correlation with a person having one trait versus another.

9 | Head and Neck Anatomy

SHORT ANSWER QUESTIONS

1. Identify the regions of the head.
2. Identify the bones of the cranium and face.
3. Locate and identify muscles of the head and neck.
4. Identify and trace routes of blood vessels of the head and neck.
5. Describe the action of the temporomandibular joint.
6. Describe locations of major and minor salivary glands.
7. Describe and locate divisions of the trigeminal nerve.

FILL IN THE BLANK

Select the best term from the list below and complete the following statements.

Abducens nerve
Ala
Anterior jugular vein
Articular space
Buccal
Circumvallate lingual papillae
Cranium
Greater palatine nerve
Hyoid bone
Infraorbital region
Lacrimal bones
Masseter muscle
Occipital region
Parotid duct
Temporomandibular disorder
Temporomandibular joint
Salivary glands
Sternocleidomastoid
Trapezius
Xerostomia

1. A vein that begins below the chin, descends near the midline, and drains into the external jugular vein is the

    _____.

2. The eight bones that cover and protect the

    brain are the _____.

3. The _____ nerve serves the posterior hard palate and posterior lingual gingiva.

4. _____ refers to structures that are closest to the inner cheek.

5. Large papillae on the tongue are

    _____.

6. The _____ is the primary support for the tongue and other muscles.

7. The region of the head that is located below the orbital region is the

    _____.

8. Paired facial bones that help form the medial wall of the orbit are the

    _____.

9. The _____ is the most obvious and strongest muscle of mastication.

10. The _____ is the region of the head overlying the occipital bone and covered by the scalp.

11. The _____ glands produce saliva.

12. One of the cervical muscles that divides the neck region into anterior and posterior cervical triangles is the _____.

13. The space between the capsular ligament and between the surfaces of the glenoid fossa and the condyle is the

    _____.

14. _____ is the sixth cranial nerve that serves the eye muscle.

15. _____ is a winglike cartilaginous structure of the nose.

16. A joint on each side of the head that allows for movement of the mandible is the _____.

17. _____ is a disease process associated with the temporomandibular joint.

18. The _____ is one of the cervical muscles that lifts the clavicle and scapula when you shrug your shoulder.

19. _____ is a term for decreased production of saliva.

20. The _____ is associated with the parotid salivary gland that opens into the oral cavity at the parotid papilla.

MULTIPLE CHOICE

Complete each question by circling the best answer.

1. The regions of the head include the frontal, parietal, occipital, temporal, orbital, nasal, infraorbital, and:

   a. mandible.
   b. maxilla.
   c. zygomatic.
   d. lacrimal.

2. What bone forms the forehead?

   a. Occipital
   b. Frontal
   c. Parietal
   d. Zygomatic

3. What bone forms the back and base of the cranium?

   a. Parietal
   b. Temporal
   c. Occipital
   d. Frontal

4. Which bones form the cheek?

   a. Sphenoid
   b. Zygomatic
   c. Temporal
   d. Nasion

5. Which bones form the upper jaw and hard palate?

   a. Zygomatic
   b. Sphenoid
   c. Mandible
   d. Maxilla

6. Name the only movable bone of the skull.

   a. Coronoid process
   b. Temporal
   c. Mandible
   d. Maxilla

7. Where is the mental foramen located?

   a. Maxilla
   b. Coronoid process
   c. Mandible
   d. Glenoid process

8. What are the basic types of movement by the TMJ?

   a. Up and down
   b. Hinge and glide
   c. Side to side
   d. Back and forth

9. What type of symptom may a patient who is experiencing TMD exhibit?

   a. Migraine
   b. Nausea
   c. Temperature
   d. Pain

10. Which cranial nerve innervates all muscles of mastication?

   a. Third
   b. Fourth
   c. Fifth
   d. Sixth

11. What is the name of the horseshoe-shaped bone where muscles of the tongue and the floor of the mouth attach?

   a. Hyoid
   b. Sphenoid
   c. Mandible
   d. Vomer

12. Which of the major salivary glands is the largest?

   a. Submandibular
   b. Sublingual
   c. Parotid
   d. Submaxillary

13. What is another name for the parotid duct?

    a. Ducts of Rivinus
    b. von Ebner's
    c. Wharton's duct
    d. Stensen's duct

14. Give the artery that is behind the ramus and branches along the mandible.

    a. Infraorbital artery
    b. Facial artery
    c. Inferior alveolar artery
    d. Lingual artery

15. Which artery supplies the maxillary molars, premolar teeth, and gingiva?

    a. Inferior alveolar artery
    b. Posterior superior alveolar artery
    c. Facial artery
    d. Lingual artery

16. How many pairs of cranial nerves are connected to the brain?

    a. 4 pairs
    b. 6 pairs
    c. 10 pairs
    d. 12 pairs

17. Which division of the trigeminal nerve subdivides into the buccal, lingual, and interior alveolar nerves?

    a. Mandibular division
    b. Facial division
    c. Lingual division
    d. Maxillary division

18. During what type of dental examination would lymph nodes be palpated?

    a. Physical exam
    b. Intraoral exam
    c. Extraoral exam
    d. Radiographic exam

19. What is the term for enlarged or palpable lymph nodes?

    a. Lymphadenopathy
    b. Xerostomia
    c. Parkinson's disease
    d. Lymphitis

CASE STUDY

One of the most important responsibilities of the clinical assistant is to control moisture during a dental procedure. Moisture can contaminate the operative site, prevent a dental material from setting, and even be the cause for having to start over.

1. What kind of moisture could interfere with a dental procedure?
2. How is saliva produced?
3. Locate where in the mouth saliva would be produced.
4. Describe ways that you can control moisture during a procedure.

10 | Landmarks of the Face and Oral Cavity

SHORT ANSWER QUESTIONS

1. Name and identify the landmarks of the face.
2. Name and identify the landmarks of the oral cavity.
3. Describe the structures found in the vestibule region of the oral cavity.
4. Describe the area of the oral cavity proper.
5. Describe the characteristics of normal gingival tissue.
6. Match each sensation of taste to the specific region of the tongue.

FILL IN THE BLANK

Select the best term from the list below and complete the following statements.

Ala of the nose
Anterior naris
Canthus
Commissure
Fordyce's spots
Gingiva
Glabella
Labial frenum
Mental protuberance
Nasion
Philtrum
Septum
Tragus of the ear
Vermilion border
Vestibule

1. _____ is the fold of tissue at the corner of the eyelids.

2. The winglike tip of the outer side of each nostril is the _____.

3. The _____ is the rectangular area from under the nose to the midline of the upper lip.

4. _____ is the cartilage projection anterior to the external opening of the ear.

5. The _____ is the midpoint between the eyes, just below the eyebrows.

6. _____ is the smooth surface of the frontal bone directly above the root of the nose.

7. The tissue that divides the nasal cavity into two nasal fossae is the _____.

8. _____ is also known as the nostril.

9. The part of the mandible that forms the chin is the _____.

10. The _____ is the darker-colored border around the lips.

11. The _____ is the angle at the corner of the mouth where the upper and lower lips join.

12. The space between the teeth and the inner mucosal lining of the lips and cheeks is the _____.

13. _____ are normal variations that sometimes appear on the buccal mucosa.

14. The _____ is a band of tissue that passes from the facial oral mucosa at the midline of the arch to the midline of the inner surface of the lip.

15. Masticatory mucosa that covers the alveolar processes of the jaws and surrounds the necks of the teeth is the

_____.

MULTIPLE CHOICE

Complete each question by circling the best answer.

1. What region of the face extends from the eyebrows to the hairline?

    a. Temple
    b. Zygomatic malar
    c. Forehead
    d. Nose

2. The line that marks a color change from your face to your lips is referred to as the:

    a. commissure.
    b. vermilion border.
    c. fordyce.
    d. labial frenum.

3. What type of tissue covers the oral cavity?

    a. Mucous membrane
    b. Epithelial
    c. Squamous
    d. Stratified

4. Besides the oral cavity proper, give the other region of the oral cavity.

    a. Gingiva
    b. Tongue
    c. Lips
    d. Vestibule

5. The structure that passes from the oral mucosa to the facial midline of the mandibular arch is the:

    a. tongue.
    b. frenum.
    c. uvula.
    d. incisive papilla.

6. What is the proper term for your patient's gums?

    a. Epithelia
    b. Incisive
    c. Skin
    d. Gingiva

7. What is another term for unattached gingiva?

    a. Interdental gingiva
    b. Gingival groove
    c. Free gingiva
    d. Attached gingiva

8. Another term for the interdental gingivae is:

    a. papilla.
    b. gingival groove.
    c. free gingiva.
    d. attached gingiva.

9. What is the name of the pear-shaped pad of tissue behind the maxillary incisors?

    a. Palatine rugae
    b. Incisive papilla
    c. Palatine raphe
    d. Uvula

10. What is the name of the hanging projection of tissue at the border of the soft palate?

    a. Palatine rugae
    b. Free gingiva
    c. Uvula
    d. Incisive papilla

11. What is the correct term for the upper surface of the tongue?

    a. Frontal
    b. Dorsum
    c. Ventral
    d. Apex

12. The thin fold of mucous membrane that extends from the floor of the mouth to the underside of the tongue is the:

    a. sublingual fold.
    b. sublingual caruncle.
    c. lingual frenum.
    d. incisive frenum.

CASE STUDY

Almost every skin product that we use today has some type of skin safeguard from the harmful rays of the sun. As health care providers, it is our responsibility to educate our patients with health news and new products and techniques.

1. What type of harmful rays does the sun give off?
2. Why would a dental team discuss facial and skin concerns with a patient?
3. What specific areas of the face would be most susceptible to sun damage?
4. Describe products that you could recommend to a patient for specific areas of the face to help block out harmful rays from the sun.

11 | Overview of the Dentition

SHORT ANSWER QUESTIONS

1. Explain how the size and shape of teeth determine their functions.
2. Describe the various functions of each type of teeth.
3. Name and identify the location of each of the tooth surfaces.
4. Explain the differences between primary, mixed, and permanent dentition.
5. Define occlusion, centric occlusion, and malocclusion.
6. Name and describe Angle's classification of malocclusion.
7. Name and describe the three primary systems of tooth numbering.

FILL IN THE BLANK

Select the best term from the list below and complete the following statements.

Anterior
Centric occlusion
Curve of Spee
Deciduous
Dentition
Embrasures
Functional occlusion
Interproximal space
Malocclusion
Mandibular arch
Masticatory surface
Maxillary arch
Occlusion
Posterior
Quadrant
Sextant
Succedaneous teeth

1. Natural teeth in the dental arch are your _____.

2. _____ are called baby or primary teeth.

3. The natural contact of the maxillary and mandibular teeth in all positions is your _____.

4. Permanent teeth that replace primary teeth are _____.

5. The upper jaw is your _____.

6. The lower jaw is your _____.

7. A(n) _____ is one fourth of the dentition.

8. A(n) _____ is one sixth of the dentition.

9. _____ means toward the front.

10. _____ means toward the back.

11. The chewing surface of the teeth is the _____.

12. _____ is the area between adjacent tooth surfaces.

13. A(n) _____ is a triangular space in the gingival direction between the proximal surfaces of two adjoining teeth in contact.

14. Your teeth are in _____ when there is maximum contact between the occluding surfaces of the maxillary and mandibular teeth.

15. Teeth are in _____ when the contact of the teeth occlude during biting and chewing movements.

16. _____ is an abnormal or malpositioned relationship of the maxillary teeth to mandibular teeth when they are in centric occlusion.

17. The _____ is the curvature formed by the maxillary and mandibular arches in occlusion.

MULTIPLE CHOICE

Complete each question by circling the best answer.

1. Name the two sets of teeth humans have in their lifetime.

    a. Secondary
    b. Primary
    c. Permanent
    d. b and c

2. How many teeth are in the primary dentition?

    a. 10
    b. 20
    c. 28
    d. 32

3. What is the term for the four sections of the divided dental arches?

    a. Sextant
    b. Maxillary
    c. Mandibular
    d. Quadrant

4. What term is used for the front teeth?

    a. Maxillary
    b. Anterior
    c. Mandibular
    d. Posterior

5. Name the most posterior teeth.

    a. Centrals
    b. Laterals
    c. Premolars
    d. Molars

6. Which tooth is known as the cornerstone of the dental arch?

    a. Lateral
    b. Central
    c. Canine
    d. Molar

7. Name the surface of the tooth facing the tongue.

    a. Lingual
    b. Facial
    c. Mesial
    d. Distal

8. What is the name for the space between adjacent teeth?

    a. Occlusion
    b. Bite
    c. Interproximal
    d. Facial

9. The name of the area where adjacent teeth physically touch is the:

    a. embrasure.
    b. contact area.
    c. occlusion.
    d. interproximal.

10. The name of the triangular space between adjacent teeth is the:

    a. embrasure.
    b. contact area.
    c. occlusion.
    d. interproximal.

11. The junction of two teeth surfaces is a(n):

    a. margin.
    b. proximal surface.
    c. angle.
    d. pit.

12. What third of the surface of a tooth is toward the end of the root?

    a. Occlusal third
    b. Middle third
    c. Apical third
    d. Proximal third

13. The term for the position of teeth during chewing is:

    a. functional occlusion.
    b. malocclusion.
    c. mastication.
    d. distocclusion.

14. A person who has an incorrect bite is diagnosed with:

    a. functional occlusion.
    b. malocclusion.
    c. mastication.
    d. neutrocclusion.

15. What is the technical term for Class III occlusion?

    a. Functional occlusion
    b. Distocclusion
    c. Malocclusion
    d. Mesiocclusion

16. What classification is neutrocclusion?

    a. Class I
    b. Class II
    c. Class III
    d. Class IV

17. What is the name for the arch of the occlusal plane?

    a. Curve of occlusion
    b. Curve of Spee
    c. Curve of molars
    d. Curve of Ortho

CASE STUDY

While assisting the dentist in an intraoral examination, the dentist has asked you to record the existing teeth using the Universal system. Beside each tooth indicate its Universal number.

Maxillary right second molar
Maxillary right first molar
Maxillary right first premolar
Maxillary right canine
Maxillary right lateral
Maxillary right central
Maxillary left central
Maxillary left canine
Maxillary left second premolar
Maxillary left first molar
Maxillary left third molar
Mandibular left second molar
Mandibular left first molar
Mandibular left canine
Mandibular left lateral
Mandibular left central
Mandibular right central
Mandibular right canine
Mandibular right second premolar
Mandibular right second molar

12 | Tooth Morphology

SHORT ANSWER QUESTIONS

1. Identify each tooth using the correct name.
2. Describe the general and specific features of each tooth in the permanent dentition.
3. Discuss clinical considerations of each tooth in the permanent dentition.
4. Describe the general and specific features of the primary dentition.
5. Discuss clinical considerations with the primary dentition.

FILL IN THE BLANK

Select the best term from the list below and complete the following statements.

Canine eminence
Central groove
Cingulum
Cusp
Fossa
Furcation
Imbrication lines
Incisal edge
Inclined cuspal planes
Mamelon
Marginal ridge
Morphology
Nonsuccedaneous

1. The _____ is a major elevation on the masticatory surface of canines and permanent teeth.

2. A wide, shallow depression on the lingual surface of anterior teeth is the

   _____.

3. _____ is an area between two or more root branches.

4. _____ is the external vertical bony ridge on the facial surface of the canines.

5. The most prominent developmental groove on posterior teeth is the _____.

6. The _____ is a raised, rounded area on the cervical third of the lingual surface.

7. Slight ridges that run mesiodistally in the cervical third of teeth are

   _____.

8. The rounded enamel extension on the incisal ridge of incisors is the _____.

9. A rounded, raised border on the mesial and distal portions of the lingual surface of anterior teeth and the occlusal table of posterior teeth is the _____.

10. A ridge on the permanent molars that appears flattened on labial, lingual, or incisal view after tooth eruption is the

    _____.

11. _____ are the sloping areas between the cusp ridges.

12. _____ refers to a tooth that does *not* replace a primary tooth.

13. _____ is the study of the form and shape of teeth.

MULTIPLE CHOICE

Complete each question by circling the best answer.

1. How many anterior teeth are in the permanent dentition?

   a. 10
   b. 12
   c. 28
   d. 32

2. What term is given to a permanent tooth that replaces a primary tooth of the same type?

   a. Implant
   b. Crown
   c. Succedaneous
   d. Molar

3. What is the rounded, raised area on the cervical third of the lingual surface of anterior teeth?

   a. Cingulum
   b. Mamelon
   c. Ridge
   d. Edge

4. What feature do newly erupted central and lateral incisors have on their incisal ridge?

   a. Cingulum
   b. Mamelon
   c. Ridge
   d. Cusp

5. Which teeth are the longest ones in the permanent dentition?

   a. Molar
   b. Central incisor
   c. Premolar
   d. Canine

6. Which teeth are the smallest ones in the permanent dentition?

   a. Maxillary molars
   b. Maxillary laterals
   c. Mandibular premolars
   d. Mandibular centrals

7. What is the name for the developmental horizontal lines on anterior teeth?

   a. Imbrication lines
   b. Marginal lines
   c. Oblique lines
   d. Incisal lines

8. What feature borders the occlusal table of a posterior tooth?

   a. Oblique ridges
   b. Triangular ridges
   c. Marginal ridges
   d. Incisal ridges

9. What is the pinpoint depression where two or more grooves meet?

   a. Fossa
   b. Sulcus
   c. Ridge
   d. Pit

10. Which teeth are frequently extracted as part of orthodontic treatment?

    a. Lateral incisors
    b. First premolars
    c. Third molars
    d. Canines

11. What occlusal form does the mandibular second premolar appear like?

    a. Incisal edge
    b. Two cusps
    c. Three cusps
    d. b and c

12. What term is given to a tooth with three roots?

    a. Furcation
    b. Bifurcation
    c. Trifurcation
    d. Quadrifuraction

13. What term is given to a tooth that does *not* replace a primary tooth?

    a. Succedaneous
    b. Nonsuccedaneous
    c. Supernumerary
    d. Developmental

14. What is the name of the fifth cusp on a maxillary first molar?

    a. Cingulum
    b. Fossa
    c. Mamelon
    d. Cusp of Carabelli

15. How many roots do mandibular molars have?

    a. One root
    b. Two roots
    c. Three roots
    d. b or c

16. Which teeth are referred to as wisdom teeth?

    a. Central incisors
    b. Canines
    c. First molars
    d. Third molars

17. How dense is the enamel covering on a primary tooth?

    a. Thin
    b. Medium
    c. Thick
    d. Double that of a permanent tooth

18. What method of identification is used in the Universal Tooth Numbering System for the primary dentition?

    a. Numerical
    b. Italicized
    c. Alphabetical
    d. Pictorial

19. Which primary tooth has an H-shaped groove pattern on its occlusal surface?

    a. Maxillary premolar
    b. Mandibular molar
    c. Maxillary premolar
    d. Maxillary molar

20. Which primary tooth is the largest?

    a. Maxillary central
    b. Mandibular molar
    c. Maxillary molar
    d. Mandibular canine

CASE STUDY

You have been assigned a project in your dental anatomy class. You are assigned to carve a maxillary first molar from wax.

1. Which specific features will you include in the anatomical crown of your carving?
2. How many cusps will you carve?
3. What type of ridges will you carve onto the occlusal surface?
4. How many roots will you carve?
5. How will the roots be positioned from the crown?

13 | Dental Caries

SHORT ANSWER QUESTIONS

1. Explain the process of dental caries.
2. Name the risk factors for dental caries.
3. Explain the purpose of caries activities tests.
4. Discuss the modes of transmission of dental caries.
5. Identify the infective agent in the caries process.
6. Explain the role of saliva in oral health.
7. Explain the cause and effect of diet and dental caries.
8. Explain the remineralization process.
9. List the differences between root caries and smooth surface caries.
10. Discuss the advantages and disadvantages of the laser caries detection device.

FILL IN THE BLANK

Select the best term from the list below and complete the following statements.

Caries
Cavitation
Demineralization
Fermentable carbohydrates
Incipient caries
Lactobacillus
Mutans streptococci
Pellicle
Plaque
Rampant caries
Remineralization
Xerostomia

1. Another name for tooth decay is

   _____.

2. _____ is the loss of minerals from the tooth.

3. _____ is the replacement of minerals in the tooth.

4. The type of bacteria primarily responsible for caries is _____.

5. _____ is a type of bacteria that produces lactic acid from carbohydrates.

6. _____ is a colorless, sticky mass of microorganisms that adheres to teeth surfaces.

7. The formation of a cavity or hole is

   _____.

8. _____ is the beginning or coming into existence.

9. Decay that develops rapidly and is widespread throughout the mouth is

   termed _____.

10. _____ is dryness of the mouth caused by abnormal reduction in the amount of saliva.

11. A thin coating of salivary materials that is deposited on tooth surfaces is

    _____.

12. Simple carbohydrates such as sucrose, fructose, lactose, and glucose are

    _____.

MULTIPLE CHOICE

Complete each question by circling the best answer.

1. The bacteria that cause dental caries are:

   a. spirochetes.
   b. mutans streptococci.
   c. staphylococci.
   d. monocytes.

2. What is the soft, sticky, bacterial mass that adheres to teeth?

   a. Decay
   b. *Lactobacillus*
   c. Plaque
   d. Carbohydrates

3. What mineral in the enamel makes the crystal easier to dissolve?

    a. Carbonated apatite
    b. Iron
    c. Calcium
    d. Magnesium

4. The three factors necessary for the formation of dental caries are bacteria, fermentable carbohydrates, and:

    a. saliva.
    b. poor toothbrushing habits.
    c. susceptible tooth.
    d. nonfluoridated water.

5. What is the term for the dissolving of calcium and phosphate from a tooth?

    a. Demineralization
    b. Resorption
    c. Remineralization
    d. Absorption

6. A patient with rapid and extensive formation of caries is diagnosed with:

    a. malocclusion.
    b. xerostomia.
    c. rampant caries.
    d. TMD.

7. Caries that occurs under or adjacent to existing dental restorations is diagnosed as:

    a. gingivitis.
    b. periodontitis.
    c. rampant caries.
    d. recurrent caries.

8. How does saliva protect the teeth from dental caries?

    a. Physical actions
    b. Chemical actions
    c. Antibacterial actions
    d. All of the above

CASE STUDY

Jeramy Allen is a 13-year-old patient of the practice. To date he has had nine restorations and is scheduled to come back to have another restoration placed. In reviewing his patient record, you notice that most of his restorations are on the chewing surface of his teeth.

1. Is it normal for a 13-year-old to have this many restorations?
2. What might be causing Jeramy to have a high rate of caries?
3. What dental term describes the surface of his teeth that have restorations?
4. Where in the patient record could you locate such information?
5. How can you educate Jeramy to help reduce his rate of caries?

14 | Periodontal Diseases

SHORT ANSWER QUESTIONS

1. Name and describe the tissues of the periodontium.
2. Identify and describe the two main types of periodontal diseases.
3. Explain the significance of plaque and calculus in relation to periodontal disease.
4. List and describe the American Academy of Periodontology case types of periodontal disease.
5. Describe the two types of calculus.
6. Identify three causes of gingivitis.
7. Identify three types of periodontitis.

FILL IN THE BLANK

Select the best term from the list below and complete the following statements.

Calculus
Gingivitis
Periodontal diseases
Periodontitis
Periodontium
Plaque
Subgingival
Supragingival

1. A soft deposit on teeth that consists of bacteria and bacterial byproducts is

   _____.

2. _____ is made up of calcium and phosphate salts in saliva that become mineralized and adhere to tooth surface.

3. The _____ are those structures that surround, support, and are attached to the teeth.

4. Diseases of the periodontium are

   _____.

5. _____ refers to the area above the gingiva.

6. _____ refers to the area below the gingiva.

7. Inflammation of the gingival tissue is

   _____.

8. _____ is an inflammatory disease of the supporting tissues of the teeth.

MULTIPLE CHOICE

Complete each question by circling the best answer.

1. Gingivitis is an:

   a. inflammation of the periodontium.
   b. inflammation of the alveolar process.
   c. inflammation of the gingiva.
   d. inflammation of the oral mucosa.

2. A clinical sign of gingivitis is:

   a. caries.
   b. redness.
   c. temperature.
   d. ulcers.

3. What can be done to reverse gingivitis?

   a. Improve brushing and flossing techniques
   b. Take antibiotics
   c. Root planing
   d. Fluoride treatment

4. Periodontitis is an:

   a. inflammation of the periodontium.
   b. inflammation of the alveolar process.
   c. inflammation of the gingiva.
   d. inflammation of the oral mucosa.

5. How many basic case types of periodontal disease are recognized?

   a. two
   b. three
   c. four
   d. five

CASE HISTORY

Sally Hunter is 14 years old and wears braces. She has returned to the orthodontist for her 6-week check. While evaluating her braces, you notice that her gingiva is red, and slightly inflamed. You look back at her patient record, and there is no indication of this at her last check.

1. To what would you attribute this gingival appearance?
2. Could there be any other reason that Sally's gingival tissue would be this way?
3. Where in the patient record would this be noted if her gingiva was like this before?
4. What diagnosis would Sally be given for the appearance of her gingiva?
5. How can this problem be alleviated?

15 | Preventive Dentistry

SHORT ANSWER QUESTIONS

1. Explain the goal of preventive dentistry.
2. Name and describe the components of a preventive dentistry program.
3. Describe the key components of preventive dentistry.
4. Identify sources of systemic fluoride.
5. Discuss techniques for educating patients in preventive care.
6. Name and discuss three methods of fluoride therapy.
7. Describe the effects of excessive amounts of fluoride.
8. Describe the purpose of a fluoride needs assessment.
9. Compare and contrast the methods of toothbrushing.
10. Describe the process for cleaning a denture.

FILL IN THE BLANK

Select the best term from the list below and complete the following statements.

Dental sealants
Disclosing agent
Preventive dentistry
Systemic fluoride
Topical fluoride

1. _____ involves patient education, the use of fluorides, dental sealants, proper nutrition, and a plaque control program.

2. _____ is a coloring agent that when applied to teeth makes plaque visible.

3. A coating that covers the occlusal pits and fissures is _____.

4. Fluoride that is ingested and then circulated through the body is _____.

5. _____ is fluoride that is applied directly to the teeth.

MULTIPLE CHOICE

Complete each question by circling the best answer.

1. What is the goal of preventive dentistry?

   a. To save money
   b. To limit visits to the dentist
   c. To have a healthy mouth
   d. To avoid having to get dental insurance

2. What is one of the most common dental diseases?

   a. Crooked teeth
   b. Dental caries
   c. Missing teeth
   d. Impacted teeth

3. What is the goal of a patient education program?

   a. To teach patients how to take care of their teeth
   b. To eliminate visits to the dentist
   c. To teach patients how to educate family members
   d. To save money on dental bills

4. What is the initial step in a patient education program?

   a. Insurance approval
   b. Intraoral examination
   c. Listening to the patient
   d. X-rays

5. Dental sealants:

   a. take the place of restorations.
   b. hold restorative materials in place.
   c. are a type of desensitizer.
   d. are a hard covering placed in the pits and fissures of teeth.

6. How does fluoride prevent decay?

   a. Demineralization
   b. Seals the teeth
   c. Remineralization
   d. a and c

7. What technique is used in the dental office to provide a fluoride treatment?

   a. Ingestion
   b. Topical
   c. Systemic
   d. Intravenous

8. What dental condition is the result of too much fluoride?

   a. Caries
   b. Gingivitis
   c. Fluorosis
   d. Periodontitis

9. What precaution is necessary for children using fluoridated toothpaste?

   a. Not to swallow the toothpaste
   b. Drink water after brushing
   c. Use only before bedtime
   d. Use only twice a day

10. What is the key dietary factor that relates to dental caries?

    a. Proteins
    b. Fats
    c. Carbohydrates
    d. Sugar

11. What information must a patient include in a food diary?

    a. Time the food was eaten
    b. Quantity
    c. Amount of sugar that was added
    d. All of the above

12. How do sugar-free sodas relate to dental caries?

    a. Decrease the acidity
    b. Increase the saliva production
    c. Increase the acidity
    d. Decrease the saliva production

13. What can patients do daily to remove plaque?

    a. Brush
    b. Rinse with water
    c. Floss
    d. a and c

14. Which type of toothbrush bristles are usually recommended?

    a. Soft
    b. Medium
    c. Hard
    d. Natural

15. Which method of toothbrushing is generally recommended?

    a. Modified Stillman
    b. Modified Bass
    c. Circular
    d. Back and forth

16. What is dental tape?

    a. Oral irrigation dental aid
    b. Flat-type interproximal dental aid
    c. Rounded-type interproximal dental aid
    d. Used for removal of calculus

17. What type of dental floss is more effective?

    a. Flavored
    b. Waxed
    c. Unwaxed
    d. b and c

18. What can be used to clean dentures?

    a. Commercial denture cleaner
    b. Mild soap
    c. Dishwashing liquid
    d. All of the above

19. What can be used to remove calculus?

    a. Toothbrush
    b. Dental scaler
    c. Floss
    d. Tape

20. If you can't brush and floss after lunch, what should you do?

    a. Rinse with mouthwash
    b. Eat an apple
    c. Rinse with water
    d. Run your tongue around your teeth

CASE STUDY

As a clinical dental assistant, your versatility and qualifications are an asset to the general dentist, dentist specialist, and dental hygienist.

1. What types of preventive procedures would you be involved in when assisting a general dentist?
2. What types of preventive procedures would you be involved in when assisting a dental hygienist?
3. What types of specialists provide preventive care?
4. What would your role be with each of these specialists in providing this care?
5. Outside of the office, what role could you take in educating the public in preventive care?

16 | Nutrition

SHORT ANSWER QUESTIONS

1. Explain why the study of nutrition is important to the dental assistant.
2. Describe the three types of proteins.
3. List the six areas of the Food Guide Pyramid.
4. Discuss the meaning of recommended dietary allowance.
5. Describe the difference between vitamins and minerals.
6. Describe the role of carbohydrates in the daily diet.
7. Explain the need for minerals in the diet.
8. Recognize the signs of eating disorders.
9. Discuss the requirement for labeling food products
10. Explain the criteria for a food to be considered organically grown.

FILL IN THE BLANK

Select the best term from the list below and complete the following statements.

Amino acids
Anorexia nervosa
Bulimia
Nutrients
Organic

1. Compounds in proteins used by the body to build and repair tissue are

   _____.

2. _____ is an eating disorder caused by a altered self-image.

3. An eating disorder characterized by binge eating and self-induced vomiting is

   _____.

4. _____ are organic and inorganic chemicals in food that supply energy.

5. Food products that have been grown without the use of any chemical pesticides, herbicides, or fertilizers are

   labeled _____.

MULTIPLE CHOICE

Complete each question by circling the best answer.

1. Nutrients provide a body:

   a. growth.
   b. energy.
   c. maintenance.
   d. all of the above

2. The three types of carbohydrates are simple sugars, complex carbohydrates, and:

   a. fats.
   b. proteins.
   c. fiber.
   d. water.

3. The term used for a food that is capable of causing tooth decay is:

   a. nutrient.
   b. cariogenic.
   c. vitamin.
   d. sugar.

4. What key nutrient helps build and repair the human body?

   a. Fats
   b. Vitamins
   c. Minerals
   d. Proteins

5. How many of the amino acids are essential?

   a. 2
   b. 4
   c. 8
   d. 12

6. One source of protein is:

   a. bread.
   b. nuts.
   c. pasta.
   d. apples.

7. Which systemic disease is related to excess dietary fat?

   a. Cardiovascular disease
   b. Allergies
   c. Multiple sclerosis
   d. Parkinson's disease

8. Which cholesterol is the "good cholesterol"?

   a. HDL
   b. LDL
   c. DDS
   d. ADA

9. Which type of vitamin is not destroyed by cooking and is stored in the body?

   a. Organic vitamins
   b. Water-soluble vitamins
   c. Fat-soluble vitamins
   d. Inorganic vitamins

10. Which vitamins are referred to as the B complex vitamins?

    a. Organic vitamins
    b. Water-soluble vitamins
    c. Fat-soluble vitamins
    d. Inorganic vitamins

11. Which vitamin is fat soluble?

    a. Calcium
    b. Riboflavin
    c. Vitamin D
    d. Magnesium

12. Which vitamin is water soluble?

    a. Vitamin A
    b. Vitamin C
    c. Phosphorus
    d. Sodium

13. Which nutrient is often called the forgotten nutrient?

    a. Calcium
    b. Vitamin C
    c. Iron
    d. Water

14. Which governmental agency regulates the labeling of food products?

    a. FDA
    b. U.S. Department of Agriculture
    c. ADA
    d. OSHA

15. What criteria are used to determine that a product is organically grown?

    a. Grown without the use of any chemical pesticides
    b. Grown without the use of any herbicides
    c. Grown without the use of any chemical fertilizers
    d. All of the above

16. What eating disorder is diagnosed when people starve themselves?

    a. Anorexia nervosa
    b. Fasting
    c. Bulimia
    d. Dieting

CASE STUDY

As a health care provider, you are involved in educating your patients daily in many areas of health issues. Nutrition is one of those areas that cannot be ignored. Not only will the lack of proper nutrition contribute to poor health, but it can also contribute to dental disease. The obesity of children has become an epidemic in today's society.

1. What do you think contributes to children being overweight?
2. Describe a commercial that contributes to children wanting to eat more.
3. Is there any one area of eating habits that contributes to children being overweight?
4. What should be the role of the dental team in educating families and their children?
5. How can poor nutrition habits affect a person's oral health?

17 | Oral Pathology

SHORT ANSWER QUESTIONS

1. Explain why the dental assistant needs to study oral pathology.
2. List and define the categories of diagnostic information.
3. Describe the warning symptoms of oral cancer.
4. Describe the cardinal signs of inflammation.
5. Describe the types of oral lesions.
6. Name five lesions that are associated with HIV/AIDS.
7. Describe the appearance of lesions associated with the use of smokeless tobacco.
8. Differentiate between chronic and acute inflammation.
9. Describe three conditions associated with the tongue.
10. Identify two oral conditions related to nutritional factors.
11. Recognize developmental disorders of the dentition.
12. List and define three anomalies that affect the number of teeth.
13. List and define five anomalies that affect the shape of the teeth.
14. Define, describe, and identify the developmental anomalies discussed in this chapter.
15. Describe the oral conditions of a patient suffering from bulimia.

FILL IN THE BLANK

Select the best term from the list below and complete the following statements.

Abscess
Biopsy
Candidiasis
Carcinoma
Cellulitis
Congenital disorder
Cyst
Ecchymosis
Erosion
Glossitis
Granuloma
Hematoma

Lesion
Leukemia
Leukoplakia
Lichen planus
Metastasize
Pathology
Sarcoma
Xerostomia

1. _____ is the study of disease.

2. A pathological site is considered a

   _____.

3. _____ is the wearing away of tissue.

4. A(n) _____ is a closed cell or pouch with a definite wall.

5. A(n) _____ is a localized collection of pus anywhere in the body.

6. A swelling or mass of blood collected in one area or organ is a

   _____.

7. _____ is the technical term for bruising.

8. A granular tumor or growth is a

   _____.

9. _____ is the formation of white spots or patches on the mucosa.

10. A benign, chronic disease affecting the skin and oral mucosa is _____.

11. _____ is a superficial infection caused by a yeastlike fungus.

12. _____ is the inflammation of cellular or connective tissue.

13. _____ is a general term used to describe inflammation of the tongue.

14. _____ is a malignant tumor in epithelial tissue.

15. _____ is a malignant tumor in connective tissue such as muscle or bone.

16. A malignant disease of the blood-forming organs is _____.

17. _____ is dryness of the mouth caused by reduction of saliva.

18. A disorder that is present at birth is called a(n) _____.

19. A(n) _____ is the removal of tissue from living patients for diagnostic examination.

20. _____ is the spreading of disease from one part of the body to another.

MULTIPLE CHOICE

Complete each question by circling the best answer.

1. What types of lesions are below the surface?
   a. Ulcers
   b. Plaque
   c. Blisters
   d. Bruises

2. What types of lesions extend above the surface?
   a. Ulcers
   b. Cysts
   c. Blisters
   d. Bruises

3. What types of lesions are even with the surface?
   a. Ulcers
   b. Cysts
   c. Plaque
   d. Bruises

4. Which condition appears as a white patch or area?
   a. Ulcer
   b. Candidiasis
   c. Leukoplakia
   d. Blister

5. Which of the following is an infection caused by a yeastlike fungus?
   a. Plaque
   b. Ulcer
   c. Leukoplakia
   d. Candidiasis

6. What is another term for canker sore?
   a. Aphthous ulcer
   b. Cellulitis
   c. Leukoplakia
   d. Plaque

7. What is the name of the condition in which inflammation causes severe pain and high fever?
   a. Glossitis
   b. Cellulitis
   c. Bruxism
   d. Candidiasis

8. What is the term for an inflammation of the tongue?
   a. Aphthous ulcer
   b. Bruxism
   c. Glossitis
   d. Cellulitis

9. What is the name of the condition in which a pattern on the tongue changes?
   a. Pseudomembranous
   b. Candidiasis
   c. Glossitis
   d. Geographic tongue

10. What is the name of the condition in which the body does not absorb vitamin B_{12}?
   a. Pernicious anemia
   b. Leukemia
   c. Periodontitis
   d. AIDS

11. What type of cancer affects the blood-forming organs?

    a. Carcinoma
    b. Sarcoma
    c. Leukemia
    d. Lymphoma

12. What is a common precancerous lesion among users of smokeless tobacco?

    a. Carcinoma
    b. Leukoplakia
    c. Lymphoma
    d. Leukemia

13. What is the term for a malignant lesion in the epithelial tissue of the oral cavity?

    a. Gingivitis
    b. Lymphoma
    c. Carcinoma
    d. Leukoplakia

14. What causes radiation caries?

    a. Heat
    b. Harmful rays
    c. Cold
    d. Lack of saliva

15. What is the name of the condition frequently seen on the lateral border of the tongue of patients with HIV/AIDS?

    a. Leukoplakia
    b. Kaposi's sarcoma
    c. Lymphadenopathy
    d. Herpes labialis

16. Which opportunistic infection is seen as purplish lesions on the skin or oral mucosa of patients with HIV/AIDS?

    a. Leukoplakia
    b. Kaposi's sarcoma
    c. Lymphadenopathy
    d. Herpes labialis

17. What is the malignant condition that involves the lymph nodes of HIV/AIDS patients?

    a. Leukoplakia
    b. Kaposi's sarcoma
    c. Lymphadenopathy
    d. Herpes labialis

18. What is the term for abnormally large jaws?

    a. Macrognathia
    b. Micrognathia
    c. Lymphoma
    d. Trismus

19. What is the name for bony growths in the palate?

    a. Periodontitis
    b. Candidiasis
    c. Hyperplasia
    d. Torus palatinus

20. What is a more common word for ankyloglossia?

    a. Lisp
    b. Cleft palate
    c. Tongue-tied
    d. Warts

21. Which dental term means tooth within a tooth?

    a. Macrognathia
    b. Dens in dente
    c. Torus
    d. Exostosis

22. Which term refers to abnormally small teeth?

    a. Anodontia
    b. Microdontia
    c. Supernumerary teeth
    d. Gemination

23. Which term describes two teeth joining together?

    a. Macrodontia
    b. Dens in dente
    c. Twinning
    d. Fusion

24. Name the hereditary abnormality in which there are hypoplasia-type defects in the enamel formation.

    a. Anodontia
    b. Ameloblastoma
    c. Amelogenesis imperfecta
    d. Dentinogenesis imperfecta

25. Name a potential complication of oral facial piercing.

    a. Infection
    b. Chipped teeth
    c. Broken teeth
    d. All of the above

CASE STUDY

Many of your patients inquire about fever blisters on their lips and inside their mouth. How would you respond to your patients when these specific questions are asked?

1. Are fever blisters from something I ate?
2. Are fever blisters affected by stress?
3. Why do I always get them on my lip?
4. What are they from?
5. Are they contagious?

18 | Microbiology

SHORT ANSWER QUESTIONS

1. Name the contributions of the early pioneers in microbiology.
2. Explain why the study of microbiology is important for the dental assistant.
3. Identify the types of bacteria according to their shape.
4. List the major groups of microorganisms.
5. Describe the differences between aerobes, anaerobes, and facultative anaerobes.
6. Identify diseases caused by chlamydias.
7. Identify the most resistant form of life known, and explain how they survive.
8. Compare viruses with bacteria, and give examples of each.
9. Discuss specificity in relation to viruses.

FILL IN THE BLANK

Select the best term from the list below and complete the following statements.

Aerobes
Anaerobes
Creutzfeldt-Jacob disease
Facultative anaerobes
Microbiology
Nonpathogenic
Oral candidiasis
Pathogenic
Prions
Protozoa
Provirus
Virulent
Viruses

1. The study of microorganisms is

    _____.

2. Disease-producing microorganisms are

    called _____.

3. _____ are microorganisms that do not produce disease.

4. _____ is capable of causing a serious disease.

5. _____ are a variety of bacteria that requires oxygen to grow.

6. Bacteria that grow in the absence of oxygen and are destroyed by oxygen are

    _____.

7. Organisms that can grow in either the presence or the absence of oxygen are

    _____.

8. A(n) _____ is a single-celled microscopic animal without a rigid cell wall.

9. _____ is a hidden virus during the latency period.

10. Ultramicroscopic infectious agents that contain either DNA or RNA are

    _____.

11. Infectious particles made up of protein that lacks nucleic acids are

    _____.

12. _____ is a rare chronic brain disease. Onset is in middle to late life (40 to 60 years).

13. _____ is a yeast infection of the oral mucosa.

MULTIPLE CHOICE

Complete each question by circling the best answer.

1. Why is microbiology important to the dental assistant?

    a. To be able to use a microscope
    b. To understand infection control
    c. To understand higher level science courses
    d. To understand the background of dental materials

2. Who is known as the Father of Microbiology?

   a. Pierre Fauchard
   b. Joseph Lister
   c. Louis Pasteur
   d. G.V. Black

3. Who was the first to record that microorganisms were responsible for hospital-acquired infections?

   a. Pierre Fauchard
   b. Joseph Lister
   c. Louis Pasteur
   d. Lucy Hobbs

4. Who was responsible for discovering the rabies vaccine?

   a. Pierre Fauchard
   b. Joseph Lister
   c. Louis Pasteur
   d. G.V. Black

5. Which is a primary shape of bacteria?

   a. Circular
   b. Rod-shaped
   c. Triangular
   d. Elongated

6. What is the name of the process for separating bacteria?

   a. Pathology test
   b. Biopsy
   c. Scratch test
   d. Gram's stain

7. What is the term for bacteria that require oxygen to grow?

   a. Aerobes
   b. Anaerobes
   c. Aerated
   d. Aerial

8. What is the most resistant form of bacterial life?

   a. Rickettsiae
   b. Virus
   c. Spores
   d. Fungi

9. How are prions different from other microorganisms?

   a. Contain only fat and one nucleic acid
   b. Contain only protein and no nucleic acids
   c. Contain no proteins and only nucleic acids
   d. Contain only carbohydrates and no phosphoric acids

CASE STUDY

There have been newspaper headlines and even announcements at your school that a severe strain of flu is going around. In class, your instructors have suggested that everyone take extra precautions to avoid getting sick.

1. How can something like the flu become an epidemic?
2. At what time of year do more people get the flu, and why?
3. If you happen to get the flu, what would your doctor most commonly prescribe?
4. Why would a special announcement be made at your school in regard to an illness?
5. Describe what you could do to avoid spreading an illness to a classmate.

19 | Disease Transmission and Infection Control

SHORT ANSWER QUESTIONS

1. Describe the differences between a chronic infection and an acute infection.
2. Describe the types of immunity and give examples of each.
3. Give an example of a latent infection.
4. Identify the links in the chain of infection.
5. Describe the methods of disease transmission in a dental office.
6. Describe the components of an OSHA Exposure Control Plan.
7. Explain the rationale for universal precautions.
8. Identify the categories of risk for occupational exposure.
9. Describe the first aid necessary following an exposure incident.
10. Discuss the rationale for HBV vaccination for dental assistants.
11. Explain the importance of hand care for dental assistants.
12. Discuss the types of necessary personal protective equipment for dental assistants.
13. Identify the various types of gloves used in a dental office.
14. Explain the types and symptoms of latex reactions.

FILL IN THE BLANK

Select the best term from the list below and complete the following statements.

Acquired immunity
Acute infection
Anaphylaxis
Artificially acquired immunity
Chronic infection
Communicable diseases
Contaminated waste
Direct contact
Droplet infection
Hazardous waste
Indirect contact
Infectious waste

Inherited immunity
Latent infection
Natural acquired immunity
Occupational exposure
OSHA Bloodborne Pathogen Standard
Percutaneous
Permucosal
Personal protective equipment
Sharps
Universal precautions

1. A persistent infection, in which the symptoms come and go, is the

   _____ period.

2. _____ infections have symptoms that are quite severe and have short duration.

3. A(n)_____ infection is of short duration.

4. The _____ was designed to protect employees against occupational exposure to bloodborne pathogens.

5. _____ is the touching or contact with a patient's blood or saliva.

6. _____ is the touching or contact with a contaminated surface or instrument.

7. A(n) _____ exposure enters the mucosal surfaces of the eyes, nose, or mouth.

8. A(n) _____ exposure enters through the skin; examples are needle sticks, cuts, and human bites.

9. A(n) _____ exposure contacts with mucous membrane, such as the eye or mouth.

10. _____ is any reasonably anticipated skin, eye, mucous membrane contact, or percutaneous injury with blood or any other potentially infectious materials.

11. The _____ is when all human blood and body fluids are to be treated as if known to be infectious with HBV, HCV, or HIV.

12. Protective clothing, masks, gloves, and eyewear for employees are considered

    _____ .

13. _____ is waste that presents a danger to humans or to the environment.

14. _____ is waste that is capable of transmitting an infectious disease.

15. Contaminated needles, scalpel blades, orthodontic wires, and endodontic instruments are considered

    _____ .

16. _____ are contaminated items that may contain the body fluids of patients, such as gloves and patient napkins.

17. The most severe form of immediate

    allergic reaction is _____ .

18. Infections that can be spread from another person or from contact with body fluids

    are _____ .

19. _____ is immunity that is present at birth.

20. _____ is immunity that is developed during a person's lifetime.

21. _____ occurs when a person has contracted and is recovering from a disease.

22. _____ occurs from a vaccination.

MULTIPLE CHOICE

Complete each question by circling the best answer.

1. What is the most common route of contamination?

   a. Air
   b. Direct contact
   c. Water
   d. Indirect contact

2. The term for acquiring an infection through mucosal tissues is:

   a. airborne.
   b. spatter.
   c. droplet infection.
   d. parenteral.

3. What infection control measures help prevent disease transmission from the dental team to the patient?

   a. Gloves
   b. Handwashing
   c. Dental dam
   d. All of the above

4. The purpose of the bloodborne pathogens standard is to:

   a. protect the patients.
   b. protect the community.
   c. protect employees.
   d. protect the Red Cross.

5. How often must the exposure control plan be reviewed and updated?

   a. Weekly
   b. Monthly
   c. Bimonthly
   d. Annually

6. Universal precautions mean:

   a. treating all patients as if they were contagious.
   b. following a universal guide on how to treat patients in the dental office.
   c. treating only patients without disease.
   d. following a specific routine in sterilization.

7. What information is included in an employee training record?

   a. Date
   b. Who conducted the training
   c. Test grade
   d. a and b

8. What must an employee do if he or she does not want the hepatitis B vaccine?

   a. Get a signature from his or her personal doctor
   b. Sign an informed consent form
   c. Have a contract drawn up by a lawyer
   d. Become certified

9. What type of soap should be used for handwashing in the dental office?

   a. Liquid antimicrobial soap
   b. Bar of antimicrobial soap
   c. Moisturizing soap
   d. Disinfectant

10. Long, artificial nails and rings should be avoided when working in a dental office because:

    a. they can stab a patient.
    b. they can scratch a patient.
    c. they can harbor pathogens.
    d. they contaminate items.

11. An example of PPE is:

    a. a dental dam.
    b. gloves.
    c. a patient napkin.
    d. a suction tip.

12. What determines the type of PPE to be worn?

    a. Risk of exposure
    b. Time of day
    c. If it is an advanced function
    d. If a patient is premedicated

13. An example of protective eyewear is:

    a. contact lenses.
    b. sunglasses.
    c. side shields.
    d. magnifying glasses.

14. What is perhaps the most critical PPE?

    a. Eyewear
    b. Mask
    c. Protective clothing
    d. Gloves

15. Sterile gloves would most commonly be worn in a:

    a. prosthodontic procedure.
    b. orthodontic procedure.
    c. surgical procedure.
    d. pediatric procedure.

16. When should utility gloves be worn?

    a. Taking out the trash
    b. Disinfecting the treatment area
    c. Preparing instruments for sterilization
    d. b and c

17. What type of gloves should be worn to open drawers during a dental procedure?

    a. Sterile
    b. Over
    c. Examination
    d. Utility

18. What is the most common type of latex allergy?

    a. Type I sensitivity
    b. Type II sensitivity
    c. Type III sensitivity
    d. Type IV sensitivity

19. What is the most serious type of latex allergic reaction?

    a. Irritant dermatitis
    b. Anaphylaxis
    c. Hay fever
    d. Asthma

20. What type of gloves should be used for a latex-sensitive patient?

    a. Over
    b. Vinyl
    c. Nitrile
    d. b and c

21. An example of contaminated waste is:

    a. patient napkins.
    b. paper towels.
    c. surface barriers.
    d. a and c

22. Another term for infectious waste is:

    a. contaminated waste.
    b. disposable waste.
    c. regulated waste.
    d. general waste.

CASE STUDY

You work in a dental office with Sheila, a dental assistant who has been in the profession for 30 years. She constantly neglects to wear PPE when working in the lab and when breaking down and disinfecting treatment rooms. Her response is that during her first 10 years as a dental assistant, she never wore PPE and was never exposed to anything.

1. Sheila has point. Why should she start wearing PPE when she didn't wear any for 10 years?
2. Why has dentistry made such a change in its standards whereas the medical community does not seem to be so strict?
3. What type of PPE should be worn when working in the lab?
4. What type of PPE should be worn when breaking down and disinfecting a treatment room?
5. How should the dentist handle this situation with Sheila?

20 | Principles and Techniques of Disinfection

SHORT ANSWER QUESTIONS

1. Explain why dental treatment room surfaces need barriers or disinfection.
2. List the types of surfaces in the dental office that are commonly covered with barriers.
3. Describe the two methods to deal with surface contamination.
4. Explain the differences between disinfection and sterilization.
5. Explain the differences between a disinfectant and an antiseptic.
6. Name the government agency that is responsible for registering disinfectants.
7. Identify chemical products commonly used for intermediate and low-level surface disinfection, and explain the advantages and disadvantages of each one.

FILL IN THE BLANK

Select the best term from the list below and complete the following statements.

Bioburden
Broad-spectrum
Chlorine dioxide
Disinfectant
Intermediate-level disinfectant
Iodophors
Low-level disinfectant
Preclean
Residual activity
Sodium hypochlorite
Splash, spatter, and droplet surfaces
Surface barrier
Synthetic phenol compounds
Touch surfaces
Tuberculocidal

1. _____ is a fluid-impervious material to cover surfaces likely to become contaminated.

2. _____ are surfaces not directly touched, but often are touched by contaminated instruments.

3. _____ are surfaces that do not contact the members of the dental team or the contaminated instruments or supplies.

4. _____ is the removal of bioburden before disinfection.

5. A chemical to reduce or lower the number of microorganisms is a

_____.

6. A(n) _____ is the action that continues long after initial application.

7. Blood, saliva, and other body fluids are

considered to be _____.

8. A(n) _____ is capable of inactivating *Mycobacterium tuberculosis*.

9. A disinfectant that is capable of killing a wide range of microbes is labeled a

_____.

10. _____ is an EPA-registered intermediate-level hospital disinfectant.

11. _____ is an EPA-registered intermediate-level hospital disinfectant with broad-spectrum disinfecting action.

12. A surface disinfectant commonly known as household bleach is _____.

13. _____ is an effective rapid-acting environmental surface disinfectant or chemical sterilant.

14. _____ destroys *M. tuberculosis*, viruses, fungi, and vegetative bacteria, and is used for disinfecting dental operatory surfaces.

15. _____ destroys certain viruses and fungi and can be used for general housecleaning purposes (e.g., walls and floors).

MULTIPLE CHOICE

Complete each question by circling the best answer.

1. Why must a surface in dental treatment rooms be disinfected or protected with barriers?

   a. To prevent injury to yourself
   b. To prevent patient-to-patient transmission of microorganisms
   c. To prevent dentist-to-patient transmission of microorganisms
   d. To prevent dental hygienist-to-assistant transmission of microorganisms

2. What is used to prevent surface contamination?

   a. Sterilization
   b. Disinfection
   c. Barriers
   d. b and c

3. What is the purpose of surface barriers?

   a. To prevent contamination
   b. To protect surface from dental materials
   c. To cover the instruments
   d. To keep water from touching the unit

4. What should you do if the barrier becomes torn?

   a. Tape it up
   b. Replace it
   c. Disinfect surface under the barrier
   d. b and c

5. Which regulation requires the use of surface disinfection?

   a. OSHA
   b. FDA
   c. ADA
   d. CDC

6. Why must surfaces be precleaned?

   a. To remove the bioburden
   b. To remove the barrier
   c. To remove spilled dental materials
   d. To remove stains

7. Which would most commonly have a barrier placed instead of being disinfected?

   a. Operator's stool
   b. Light switch
   c. Countertop
   d. Dental assistant stool

8. Where are antiseptics used?

   a. Surfaces
   b. Instruments
   c. Skin
   d. Equipment

9. Which agency regulates disinfectants?

   a. OSHA
   b. FDA
   c. ADA
   d. EPA

10. Which disinfectant is not recommended for disposable items?

    a. Glutaraldehyde
    b. Alcohol
    c. Iodophors
    d. Sodium hypochlorite

11. What is the name of the disinfectant that can leave a reddish or yellowish stain?

    a. Glutaraldehyde
    b. Alcohol
    c. Iodophors
    d. Sodium hypochlorite

12. What is a disadvantage of synthetic phenols?

    a. Stains
    b. Leave a residual film
    c. Evaporate
    d. Highly toxic

13. What is another more common term for sodium hypochlorite?

    a. Ammonia
    b. Vinegar
    c. Oil
    d. Bleach

14. Which disinfectant is not effective if blood or saliva is present?

    a. Alcohol
    b. Glutaraldehyde
    c. Chlorine dioxide
    d. Sodium hypochlorite

15. What is a common use of chlorine dioxide?

    a. Instruments
    b. Surface disinfectant
    c. Sterilant
    d. b and c

CASE STUDY

The dentist you work with has a habit of talking too much to the patients, which always puts you behind. Today you are running 30 minutes behind for the next patient, and you still have not prepared the treatment room.

1. What corners can you cut to get the room ready fast?
2. Because this scenario happens quite frequently, which would work better in this office: the use of disinfectants or the use of barriers? Why?
3. What items need to be replaced for the next patient on the dental assisting unit?
4. What items need to be replaced for the next patient on the dental unit?
5. What PPE items need to be replaced?

21 | Principles and Techniques of Sterilization

SHORT ANSWER QUESTIONS

1. Describe and discuss the seven steps of processing dental instruments.
2. Describe the three most common methods of heat sterilization, and describe the advantages and disadvantages of each.
3. Describe the precautions necessary when packaging materials for sterilization.
4. Describe the steps in sterilization of the high-speed dental handpiece.
5. Explain the differences between process indicators and process integrators.
6. Describe when and how biological monitoring is done.
7. Explain the primary disadvantage of "flash" sterilization.
8. Describe the three forms of sterilization monitoring.
9. Explain how sterilization failures can occur.
10. Explain the limitation of liquid chemical sterilants.
11. Describe the classification of instruments that determines the type of processing to be used.
12. Explain the purpose of a holding solution.
13. Describe the safety precautions necessary when operating an ultrasonic cleaner.

FILL IN THE BLANK

Select the best term from the list below and complete the following statements.

Autoclave
Biologic indicators
Biologic monitor
Chemical vapor sterilizer
Clean area
Contaminated area
Critical instrument
Dry heat sterilizer
Endospore
Noncritical instrument
Process integrator
Semicritical instrument
Sterilant
Sterilization
Ultrasonic cleaner
Use-life

1. A process that kills all microorganisms is

   _____.

2. _____ is an agent capable of killing all microorganisms.

3. The _____ is an instrument used for sterilizing by means of moist heat under pressure.

4. _____ are vials or strips, also known as spore tests, that contain harmless bacterial spores and are used to determine if sterilization has occurred.

5. The _____ is an instrument used for sterilizing by means of hot formaldehyde vapors under pressure.

6. An item used to penetrate soft tissue or bone is identified as a _____.

7. An item that comes in contact with oral tissues but does not penetrate soft tissue or bone is identified as a

   _____.

8. A(n) _____ is an item that comes in contact with intact skin only.

9. The _____ of the sterilization center is where sterilized instruments, fresh disposable supplies, and prepared trays are stored.

10. The _____ of the sterilization center is where contaminated items are brought for precleaning.

11. An instrument used for sterilization by means of heated air is the

    _____.

12. _____ is the period of time that a germicidal solution is effective after it has been prepared for use.

13. The _____ verifies sterilization by confirming that all spore-forming microorganisms have been destroyed.

14. Tapes, strips, or tabs with heat-sensitive chemicals that change color when exposed to a certain temperature are the

    _____.

15. A(n) _____ is a resistant, dormant structure, formed inside of some bacteria, that can withstand adverse conditions

16. The _____ is an instrument that loosens and removes debris by sound waves traveling through a liquid.

MULTIPLE CHOICE

Complete each question by circling the best answer.

1. The instrument classifications used to determine the method of sterilization are:

   a. critical.
   b. semicritical.
   c. noncritical.
   d. all of the above

2. What type of personal protective equipment is necessary when processing instruments?

   a. Goggle-type eyewear
   b. Sterile gloves
   c. Surgical scrubs
   d. Hairnet

3. The basic rule of the workflow pattern in an instrument processing area is:

   a. triangular.
   b. square.
   c. linear.
   d. circular.

4. If instruments cannot be processed immediately, what should be done with them?

   a. Kept in the dental treatment area
   b. Wrapped in aluminum foil
   c. Covered with a patient napkin
   d. Placed in a holding solution

5. How are instruments precleaned?

   a. Hand scrubbing
   b. Ultrasonic cleaning
   c. Thermal washer/disinfector
   d. All of the above

6. Which method of precleaning instruments is the *least* desirable?

   a. Hand scrubbing
   b. Ultrasonic cleaning
   c. Thermal washer
   d. Microwave

7. The ultrasonic cleaner works:

   a. by microwaves.
   b. by sound waves.
   c. by ultraviolet waves.
   d. by light waves.

8. Why can't kitchen dishwashers be used to preclean instruments?

   a. Not ADA approved
   b. Not CDC approved
   c. Not FDA approved
   d. Not OSHA approved

9. How can the rusting of instruments be prevented?

   a. Use of a disinfectant
   b. Use of lubrication
   c. Use of proper wrapping
   d. Use of wax

10. Why should instruments be packaged for sterilization?

    a. Maintain sterility
    b. For identification
    c. Maintain organization
    d. For pre-setup

11. Why are pins, staples, or paper clips not used on instrument packaging?

    a. Become too hot to touch
    b. Cannot record information on the package
    c. Damage the sterilizer
    d. Cause holes in the packaging

12. Which is a form of sterilization monitoring?

    a. Physical
    b. Chemical
    c. Biological
    d. All of the above

13. Where do you place a process indicator?

    a. Inside of package
    b. Outside of package
    c. Inside of sterilizer
    d. Outside of sterilizer

14. Where do you place a process integrator?

    a. Inside of package
    b. Outside of package
    c. Inside of sterilizer
    d. Outside of sterilizer

15. Do process indicators and integrators assure that an item is sterile?

    a. Yes
    b. No

16. What is the best way to determine if sterilization has occurred?

    a. Check the sterilizer
    b. Process indicator
    c. Through biological monitoring
    d. Process integrator

17. What causes sterilization failures?

    a. Improper contact of sterilizing agent
    b. Improper temperature
    c. Improper sterilizer
    d. a and b

18. What are the most commonly used forms of heat sterilization?

    a. Steam
    b. Chemical vapor
    c. Dry heat
    d. All of the above

19. What is a primary disadvantage of "flash" sterilization?

    a. Type of sterilizer
    b. Inability to wrap items
    c. Temperature
    d. Sterilizing agent used

20. What is a major advantage of chemical vapor sterilization?

    a. Sterilizing time is faster
    b. Sterilize more instruments at one time
    c. Will not rust instruments
    d. Do not have to wrap the instruments

21. An example of dry heat sterilization is:

    a. chemical vapor.
    b. autoclave.
    c. microwave.
    d. static air.

22. What is the primary disadvantage of liquid chemical sterilization?

    a. Cannot perform biological monitoring
    b. No heat involved
    c. Cannot wrap instruments
    d. Not a closed environment

23. How are instruments rinsed that have been processed in a liquid chemical sterilant?

    a. With hot water
    b. With cold water
    c. With sterile water
    d. With carbonated water

24. How is the high-speed handpiece prepared for sterilization?

    a. Placed in a holding bath
    b. Flushed
    c. Soaked in soapy water
    d. Taken apart

25. What type of heat sterilization is appropriate for high-speed handpieces?

    a. Steam
    b. Chemical vapor
    c. Liquid chemical sterilant
    d. a and b

CASE STUDY

You are the only clinical assistant in the practice, and your morning has been very hectic. None of the contaminated instruments have been processed for the afternoon. When you finally get a break and get back to the sterilization center, your dirty instruments are in the ultrasonic and the trays and paper products are on the counter.

1. How could this backup of instruments been prevented?
2. You have five trays of instruments in the ultrasonic. Now what?
3. Is there anything that you could have done immediately after a procedure to change this circumstance?
4. Is there anyone else in the dental office who could help you process instruments? If so, how could you arrange this?
5. Should you discuss this situation with the dentist?

22 | Regulatory and Advisory Agencies

SHORT ANSWER QUESTIONS

1. Explain the difference between regulations and recommendations.
2. List four professional sources for dental information.
3. Name the premier infection control educational organization in dentistry.
4. Describe the role of the Centers for Disease Control and Prevention.
5. Explain a primary difference between OSHA and NIOSH.
6. Describe the role of the Environmental Protection Agency in relation to dentistry.
7. Describe the role of the Food and Drug Administration in relation to dentistry.

FILL IN THE BLANK

Select the best term from the list below and complete the following statements.

ADA
CDC
EPA
FDA
NIOSH
OSAP
OSHA

1. The _____ is a federal regulatory agency concerned with the regulation of sterilization equipment.

2. A federal agency that is nonregulatory and issues recommendations on health and

   safety is the _____.

3. _____ is the professional organization for dentists.

4. A federal regulatory agency that enforces regulations pertaining to employee safety is

   the _____.

5. _____ is the premier infection control education organization in dentistry.

6. _____ is a federal agency that conducts research and makes recommendations for the prevention of work-related disease and injury.

7. The _____ is a federal regulatory agency that deals with issues concerning the environment or public safety.

MULTIPLE CHOICE

Complete each question by circling the best answer.

1. What is the primary focus of the CDC in dentistry?
   a. Public health
   b. Research
   c. Drugs
   d. Employees

2. What is the primary focus of the FDA in dentistry?
   a. Research
   b. Public health
   c. Drugs
   d. Employees

3. What is the primary focus of the EPA in dentistry?
   a. Research
   b. Public health
   c. Employees
   d. Environment

4. What is the primary focus of OSHA in dentistry?
   a. Public health
   b. Employees
   c. Environment
   d. Research

CASE STUDY

Your dentist uses many custom trays in the dental office. The material that is available for you to make these trays is acrylic resin. A friend of yours who is a dental assistant in a different practice informed you that acrylic resin is very volatile and that you should try a different kind of material.

1. What is a custom tray?
2. What does *volatile* mean?
3. Why is a material like this available if it is harmful to you?
4. Discuss the health risks of acrylic resin and how you can protect yourself when using such a material.
5. What organization would be involved in identifying the ingredients in acrylic resin that can harm the public or the environment?

23 | Chemical Safety

SHORT ANSWER QUESTIONS

1. Describe potential long- and short-term effects of exposure to chemicals.
2. Explain the components of the OSHA Hazard Communication Standard.
3. Describe three common methods of chemical exposure.
4. Describe the components of a hazard communication program.
5. Explain the purpose of a Material Safety Data Sheet.
6. Describe the difference between chronic and acute chemical exposure.
7. Identify four methods of personal protection against chemical exposure.
8. Describe how chemicals should generally be stored.
9. Discuss the recordkeeping requirements of the Hazard Communication Standard.
10. Identify types of regulated waste generated in a dental office.
11. Identify types of toxic waste generated in a dental office.
12. Discuss the packaging of regulated waste for transport.

FILL IN THE BLANK

Select the best term from the list below and complete the following statements.

Acute exposure
Chemical inventory
Chronic exposure
Contaminated waste
Environmental Protection Agency
Hazard Communication Standard
Hazardous waste
Infectious waste
Material Safety Data Sheet
Regulated waste
Toxic waste

1. The _____ is an OSHA standard regarding employees' right to know about chemicals in the workplace.

2. Forms that provide health and safety information regarding materials that contain chemicals are the

_____.

3. Repeated exposures, generally to lower levels, over a long time period are

_____.

4. _____ refers to high levels of exposure over a short period of time.

5. Waste that has certain properties or contains chemicals that could pose dangers to human health and the environment after it is discarded is

_____.

6. _____ is a comprehensive list of every product used in the office that contains chemicals.

7. The _____ is the federal agency responsible for regulating disposal of regulated waste.

8. _____ are items that have had contact with blood, saliva, or other body secretions.

9. Waste capable of causing an infectious disease is _____.

10. _____ is infectious waste that requires special handling, neutralization, and disposal.

11. Waste capable of having a poisonous effect is _____.

MULTIPLE CHOICE

Complete each question by circling the best answer.

1. What body systems could develop health-related problems as a result of exposure to chemicals?

    a. Neurological
    b. Senses
    c. Respiratory
    d. Endocrine

2. What is a primary method of chemical exposure?

    a. Inhalation
    b. Ingestion
    c. Skin contact
    d. All of the above

3. Acute chemical exposure involves:

    a. short-term exposure in large quantity.
    b. repeated exposure in small quantity.
    c. short-term exposure in smaller quantities.
    d. long-term exposure in small quantities.

4. What is a method of personal protection against chemical exposure?

    a. Ventilation
    b. Disinfected surfaces
    c. Inhalation protection
    d. Hair protection

5. What are the OSHA requirements regarding an eyewash unit?

    a. Eyewash unit in every treatment room
    b. Eyewash unit in areas where chemicals are used
    c. Eyewash unit in the building
    d. Eyewash unit on each floor

6. What could be the effects of exposure to radiographic processing solutions kept in a poorly ventilated area?

    a. Cardiac problems
    b. Reproductive problems
    c. Respiratory problems
    d. Urinary problems

7. In general, how should chemicals be stored?

    a. Cool, dry place
    b. In a locked cabinet
    c. Under water
    d. Hot, moist place

8. Chemicals are determined to be hazardous if they are:

    a. ignitable.
    b. corrosive.
    c. reactive.
    d. all of the above.

9. What is another term for the Hazard Communication Standard?

    a. Employee beware law
    b. The right-to-know law
    c. Hazardous chemical law
    d. Chemical safety law

10. What chemicals must be included in a chemical inventory?

    a. Over-the-counter drugs
    b. Prescription drugs
    c. All chemicals
    d. Dental materials

11. What is an MSDS?

    a. Material subscribed dental sheet
    b. Material safety data sheet
    c. Materials for sterilization and dental surgery
    d. Microbiology standards and disease standards

12. What materials are exempt from labeling requirements?

    a. Food
    b. Drugs
    c. Cosmetics
    d. All of the above

13. Which dental professional must receive training about hazardous chemicals?

    a. Dental laboratory technician
    b. Dental hygienist
    c. Dental assistant
    d. All of the above

14. How long must training records be kept on file?

    a. 1 year
    b. 5 years
    c. 10 years
    d. 20 years

15. An example of regulated waste is:

    a. a patient napkin.
    b. a contaminated needle.
    c. a dental dam.
    d. 2 × 2 gauze.

CASE STUDY

You have been a clinical assistant in an oral and maxillofacial surgical office for 5 years, and you teach part time in preclinic on Fridays at the dental assisting program from which you graduated. This Friday you are scheduled to work in lab with the placement of sealants. The students will be placing sealants first on extracted teeth for their check-off before they complete their practical in clinic.

1. Where did you get extracted teeth for this laboratory practical?
2. Can you save extracted teeth for such purposes?
3. How would you dispose of extracted teeth?
4. How could these teeth be prepared and used for the sealant practical?
5. If other people came to you for extracted teeth, how would you keep them for them?

24 | Dental Unit Waterlines

SHORT ANSWER QUESTIONS

1. Discuss why dental units have more bacteria than faucets do.
2. Explain the role of biofilm in dental unit waterline contamination.
3. Discuss why there is a renewed interest in dental unit waterline contamination.
4. Explain the factors in bacterial contamination of dental unit water.
5. Identify the primary source of microorganisms in dental unit water.
6. Explain the methods to reduce bacterial contamination in dental unit waterlines.

FILL IN THE BLANK

Select the best term from the list below and complete the following statements.

Biofilm
Colony-forming units
Dental unit waterlines
Legionella
Microfiltration
Planktonic bacteria
Retraction
Self-contained water reservoir

1. _____ is slime-producing bacterial communities that may also harbor fungi, algae, and protozoa.

2. The bacterium responsible for the disease legionellosis is _____.

3. _____ is the use of membrane filters to trap microorganisms suspended in water.

4. _____ are the minimum number of separable cells on the surface of a semisolid agar medium that creates a visible colony.

5. _____ consist of small-bore tubing that is usually made of plastic; they deliver dental treatment water through a dental unit.

6. A _____ is a container attached to a dental unit that is used to hold and supply water or other solutions to handpieces and air-water syringes.

7. _____ is the entry of fluids and microorganisms into waterlines as a result of negative water pressure. Also referred to as "suck back."

8. Bacteria that are floating in water are

_____.

MULTIPLE CHOICE

Complete each question by circling the best answer.

1. Are waterborne diseases limited to dentistry?

   a. Yes
   b. No

2. When was the presence of bacteria first reported in dental unit waterlines?

   a. 5 years ago
   b. 10 years ago
   c. 20 years ago
   d. 30 years ago

3. What type of public health problem is there regarding contaminated dental water?

   a. Widespread
   b. Localized
   c. No problem at this time
   d. Epidemic

4. What bacteria cause the disease legionellosis?

   a. Streptococci
   b. *Legionella* bacteria
   c. Bacilli
   d. Staphylococci

5. Where is biofilm found?

   a. Suction tips
   b. Handpiece water lines
   c. Air-water syringe water lines
   d. b and c

6. Should water be heated in the dental units to kill the bacteria?

   a. Yes
   b. No

7. Can biofilm be completely eliminated?

   a. Yes
   b. No

8. If sterile water is used in a self-contained reservoir, will the water that enters the patient's mouth be sterile?

   a. Yes
   b. No

9. How often should microfilters be changed?

   a. Daily
   b. Weekly
   c. Bimonthly
   d. Monthly

10. Which organization should you contact when selecting a chemical for the dental unit?

    a. ADA
    b. Equipment manufacturer
    c. OSHA
    d. CDC

11. What type of water must be used as an irrigant for surgery involving bone?

    a. Saline water
    b. Tap water
    c. Sterile water
    d. Carbonated water

12. Will flushing dental unit waterlines remove biofilm?

    a. Yes
    b. No

13. When should the high-volume evacuator be used to minimize aerosol?

    a. With the high-speed handpiece
    b. With the ultrasonic scaler
    c. With the air-water syringe
    d. All of the above

14. Will the use of a rubber dam totally eliminate exposure to microorganisms?

    a. Yes
    b. No

15. What type of PPE is especially critical when aerosol is being generated?

    a. Eyewear
    b. Mask
    c. Gloves
    d. a and b

CASE STUDY

A patient of the practice comments on an alarming news program that she saw last night, which showed how people could get HIV and bacterial infections from basic equipment in the dental office. She confides in you that she is not sure she wants to continue in her treatment plan.

1. Can a patient be infected with certain diseases from dental equipment?
2. What type of diseases can a patient get from dental equipment?
3. How do you respond to this patient about news shows such as these?
4. How can you alleviate your patient's fears about such instances?
5. Should the dentist be involved in this conversation?

25 | Ergonomics

SHORT ANSWER QUESTIONS

1. Describe the goal of ergonomics.
2. Discuss exercises that can reduce muscle fatigue and strengthen muscles.
3. Describe the neutral working position.
4. Describe exercises to reduce eyestrain.
5. Describe exercises to reduce neck strain.
6. Identify common symptoms of musculoskeletal disorders.
7. Identify three categories of risk factors that contribute to increased risk of injury.
8. Describe the symptoms of carpal tunnel syndrome.

FILL IN THE BLANK

Select the best term from the list below and complete the following statements.

Carpal tunnel syndrome
Cumulative trauma disorders
Ergonomics
Maximum horizontal reach
Musculoskeletal disorders
Neutral position
Normal horizontal reach
Sprains
Strains
Thenar eminence
Vertical reach

1. _____ is the adaptation of the work environment to the human body.

2. Pain resulting from ongoing stresses to muscles, tendons, nerves, and joints is

   _____.

3. _____ are disorders of the muscles and skeleton such as neck and shoulder pain, back pain, and carpal tunnel syndrome.

4. _____ is the reach created by the sweep of the forearm with the upper arm held at the side.

5. The reach created by the vertical sweep of the forearm keeping the elbow at midtorso level is _____.

6. _____ is the reach created when the upper arm is fully extended.

7. Injuries caused by extreme stretching of muscles or ligaments are

   _____.

8. _____ are injuries caused by a sudden twist or wrenching of a joint with stretching or tearing of ligaments.

9. _____ is the fleshy elevation of the palm side of the hand.

10. Pain associated with continued flexion and extension of the wrist is

    _____.

11. The _____ is the position in which the body is properly aligned and distribution of weight throughout the spine is equal.

MULTIPLE CHOICE

Complete each question by circling the best answer.

1. Ergonomics is the:

   a. prevention of air pollution.
   b. adaptation of the human body to a work environment.
   c. adaptation of the human body to an exercise routine.
   d. foundation of team dentistry.

2. The goal of ergonomics is to:

   a. learn proper exercises.
   b. help people stay healthy.
   c. perform work more effectively.
   d. b and c

3. What types of disorders are considered to be MSDs?

   a. Headaches
   b. Heartburn
   c. Eating
   d. Neurological

4. What are the risk factors that contribute to MSD injuries?

   a. Types of dental procedures
   b. Working on the maxillary arch
   c. Posture
   d. Infectious patient

5. What is neutral position?

   a. Sitting upright
   b. Weight evenly distributed
   c. Ready for instrument transfer
   d. a and b

6. A reach that is created by the sweep of your forearm with your upper arm held at your side is:

   a. normal vertical reach.
   b. normal horizontal reach.
   c. abnormal vertical reach.
   d. abnormal horizontal reach.

7. What types of gloves are most likely to aggravate carpal tunnel syndrome?

   a. Sterile gloves
   b. Overgloves
   c. Ambidextrous gloves
   d. Utility gloves

8. How can you reduce eyestrain?

   a. Prescription glasses
   b. Changing your visual distance from close up to longer distance
   c. Side shields
   d. Better lighting

9. What exercise relieves neck strain?

   a. Sit ups
   b. Jumping jacks
   c. Jogging
   d. Shoulder shrugs

10. What is one of the most important factors in preventing CTS?

    a. Resting your eyes
    b. Resting your back
    c. Resting your hands
    d. Resting your legs

CASE STUDY

You have worked with Dr. Jenkins for many years, and he has asked to meet with you today. He informs you that his eyesight has gotten so bad, that on the advice of his optometrist he must stop performing such detailed procedures. Dr. Jenkins is very distraught and does not want to give up practicing.

1. How could Dr. Jenkins's eyes have become so weakened?
2. What are some preventive measures that dental personnel can do before their eyesight gets so bad?
3. How could Dr. Jenkins still keep his practice open and refrain from detailed procedures?
4. What dental procedures would not place a lot of strain on the eyes?
5. How could you help in some of these detailed procedures?

26 | The Patient Record

SHORT ANSWER QUESTIONS

1. Describe the purpose of a patient record.
2. List the components of the patient record and describe each form.
3. Describe the importance of the patient's medical-dental health history and its relevance to dental treatment.

FILL IN THE BLANK

Select the best term from the list below and complete the following statements.

Alert
Assessment
Chronic
Chronological
Demographic
Diagnosis
Forensic dentistry
Litigation
Registration

1. _____ is the act of legal proceedings, such as a lawsuit or trial.

2. The act of evaluating a patient's conditions is known as _____.

3. A patient's illness is

   _____ if it persists over a long period of time.

4. A(n) _____ record is one that is arranged by time of occurrence.

5. _____ information relates to population, neighborhood, and race.

6. _____ is a condition or period of heightened watchfulness or preparation for action.

7. A new patient will complete a(n)

   _____ form by answering personal questions required by the dental office.

8. The process of identifying or determining the nature and cause of a disease or injury through evaluation of patient history, examination, and review of data is termed

   _____.

9. _____ is used in courts of law for the purpose of identification of an individual.

MULTIPLE CHOICE

Complete each question by circling the best answer.

1. The four things that the patient record provides are:
   a. personal information, financial status, past dentist, and the type of dental care needed.
   b. personal information, health status, types of dental care already provided, and type of dental care needed.
   c. financial status, health status, what type of dental care received, and dental care needed.
   d. personal information, health status, types of medical care already provided, and type of medical care needed.

2. What term describes the collection of data that enables the dentist to make a correct diagnosis?
   a. Assessment
   b. Decision
   c. Recall
   d. Prescription

3. The patient record is a permanent document that belongs to the:
   a. patient.
   b. dentist.
   c. court of law.
   d. dental practice.

4. Why is quality assurance so important in maintaining a practice?

    a. Describes the dental staff's qualifications
    b. Describes the dental practice's financial stability
    c. Describes the quality of care a patient is receiving
    d. Describes the dental practice's location for a specific patient population

5. How do you address a patient?

    a. By his or her first name
    b. By her maiden name
    c. By the spouse's name
    d. By his or her surname

6. Where should the patient registration form be placed?

    a. At the front of the patient record
    b. In a separate file cabinet
    c. With the charting information
    d. Behind the radiographs

7. To verify the information is accurate, what must a patient provide on the form?

    a. Date
    b. Signature
    c. Social Security number
    d. Bank deposit number
    e. a and b

8. What does the dental history section of the health history form provide for the dentist?

    a. Which procedures were legal for the dental assistant to complete
    b. Previous dental treatment and care
    c. Types of dental materials that were used
    d. Information about the previous dentist

9. Give an example of a medical alert.

    a. Has chronic arthritis
    b. Cannot be lowered in the dental chair
    c. Is allergic to specific medications
    d. Has dental insurance

CASE STUDY

Jeramy Stewart is a new patient to the practice and has been asked to come 15 minutes early to complete patient forms. After reviewing Mr. Stewart's completed forms, you recognize that he has a heart condition and is currently seeking medical care. As you go to the door to call him back to the treatment area, he inquires about a tooth that has been bothering him for a couple of weeks. You ask Mr. Stewart to have a seat, and tell him that the dentist will see him in a moment.

1. What forms would be given to a new patient to complete?
2. Should any medial alerts be indicated on the patient record? If so, what are they?
3. Should the dentist be aware of any specific details about Mr. Stewart?
4. What is your role in the examination process of a new patient?
5. What instruments and supplies did you set up for the examination of a new patient?

27 | Vital Signs

SHORT ANSWER QUESTIONS

1. List the four vital signs commonly taken in the dental office.
2. Describe how metabolism affects vital signs.
3. List the three methods described for taking a patient's temperature.
4. List the common pulse sites used in the dental office.
5. Describe characteristics of the pulse that you would look for in taking a patient's pulse.
6. Describe the characteristics of respiration and how they affect a patient's breathing.
7. Describe the best way to get accurate readings of respiration.
8. Describe the importance of taking a patient's blood pressure.
9. Differentiate the Korotkoff sounds heard during the taking of a blood pressure.

FILL IN THE BLANK

Select the best term from the list below and complete the following statements.

   Antecubital
   Arrhythmia
   Blood pressure
   Brachial
   Carotid
   Diastolic
   Electrocardiogram
   Korotkoff
   Metabolism
   Palpate
   Pulse
   Radial
   Rate
   Respiration
   Rhythm
   Sphygmomanometer
   Stethoscope
   Systolic
   Temperature
   Thermometer
   Tympanic
   Volume

1. The pressure exerted by blood against the walls of blood vessels is a person's

   _____.

2. _____ is the blood pressure reading that occurs when heart chambers are relaxed and dilated.

3. The _____ is one of the two major arteries on each side of the neck that carry blood to the head.

4. _____ relates to or resembles the arm.

5. The _____ is a record of electrical currents used in the detection and diagnosis of heart abnormalities.

6. _____ is the physical and chemical processes that occur in a living cell or organism that are necessary to maintain life.

7. An irregularity in the force or rhythm of the heartbeat is called a(n)

   _____.

8. _____ relates to the specific fold in the arm.

9. Specific sounds heard in the taking of a blood pressure are called

   _____ sounds.

10. _____ is the rhythmical throbbing of arteries produced by regular contractions of the heart.

11. _____ relates to or near the radius or forearm.

12. To examine or explore by touching is to

   _____.

13. A quantity measured is the

   _____ of something.

14. _____ is the act or process of inhaling and exhaling; breathing.

15. The instrument used for measuring blood pressure in the arteries is the

_____.

16. The instrument used for listening to sounds produced within the body is the

_____.

17. _____ is the rhythmic contraction of the heart, especially of the ventricles.

18. _____ is the degree of hotness or coldness of a body or an environment.

19. The instrument used for measuring temperature is the _____.

20. _____ is a sequence or pattern.

21. _____ relates to or resembles a drum.

22. The quantity or amount of a substance is its _____.

MULTIPLE CHOICE

Complete each question by circling the best answer.

1. The four vital signs used to detect a patient's baseline of health are:
   a. speech, temperature, gait, and electrocardiogram.
   b. height, weight, age, and race.
   c. cholesterol, blood pressure, vision, and blood sugar.
   d. respiration, temperature, pulse, and blood pressure.

2. The thermometer is used for:
   a. detecting a patient's pulse.
   b. taking a patient's temperature.
   c. reading a patient's blood pressure.
   d. counting a patient's respiration.

3. What location on the body would most commonly give the highest temperature reading of the body?
   a. Oral
   b. Ancillary
   c. Rectal
   d. Ear

4. Where is the tympanic thermometer placed?
   a. Orally
   b. Under the arm
   c. Rectally
   d. Ear

5. What artery in the body has a pulse?
   a. Carotid
   b. Radial
   c. Brachial
   d. All of the above

6. What artery would you normally palpate when taking a patient's pulse for a routine procedure?
   a. Carotid
   b. Radial
   c. Brachial
   d. Any of the above

7. The normal pulse rate for an adult is:
   a. between 25 and 65 beats.
   b. between 40 and 80 beats.
   c. between 60 and 100 beats.
   d. between 75 and 115 beats.

8. Respiration is the process of:
   a. speaking.
   b. breathing.
   c. the heart beating.
   d. walking.

9. What breathing pattern is characteristic of a very rapid rate of breathing?
   a. Bradypnea
   b. Normal
   c. Hyperventilation
   d. Sighing

10. What is the normal respiration rate for an adult?
    a. 5 to 10 breaths per minute
    b. 10 to 20 breaths per minute
    c. 18 to 30 breaths per minute
    d. 20 to 40 breaths per minute

11. What is the diastolic reading when taking a person's blood pressure?

    a. First sound heard after releasing pressure from the cuff
    b. Pulse rate taken at the brachial artery
    c. Silence between first and last sound after releasing pressure from the cuff
    d. Last sound heard after releasing pressure from the cuff

12. What instruments are used in taking a patient's blood pressure?

    a. Mouth mirror and watch with a second hand
    b. Sphygmomanometer and stethoscope
    c. Pen and paper to record reading
    d. Thermometer and electrocardiogram

13. The term for the small groove or fold on the inner arm is:

    a. antecubital.
    b. brachial.
    c. radial.
    d. femur.

14. Who discovered the series of sounds that is heard during a blood pressure reading?

    a. G.V. Black
    b. W.B. Saunders
    c. Nicolai Korotkoff
    d. C. Edmund Kells

15. The range for a normal blood pressure reading of an adult is:

    a. <90 / <60.
    b. <100 / <75.
    c. <130 / <85.
    d. <150 / <100.

CASE STUDY

Mary Robins, a 53-year-old woman, is scheduled for a routine dental prophylaxis this morning. You escort her back to the treatment area, seat her, and take her vital signs. The readings obtained today are temperature 99°, pulse 75, respirations 20, blood pressure 150/100.

1. Which dental professional would most likely be treating Mrs. Robins today?
2. Where are vital signs to be recorded?
3. Where in the dental office do you take the patient's vital signs?
4. How is a patient positioned for taking vital signs?
5. Are there any readings that are not within normal range? If so, which ones?
6. What should take place when a reading is abnormal?

28 | Oral Diagnosis and Treatment Planning

SHORT ANSWER QUESTIONS

1. List and describe the examination and diagnostic techniques for patient assessment.
2. Discuss the role of the assistant in the clinical examination.
3. List the six classifications of Black's classification of cavities.
4. Differentiate between an anatomic and a geometric diagram for charting.
5. Describe how to color code a chart diagram.
6. Describe the pocket depth and bleeding index of gingival tissues and how to record it.
7. Describe the need for a soft tissue examination.
8. Define the periodontal screening and recording (PSR) system.
9. Discuss the importance of a treatment plan.

FILL IN THE BLANK

Select the best term from the list below and complete the following statements.

Detection
Extraoral
Furcation
Intraoral
Mobility
Morphologically
Mucogingival
Palpation
Probing
Recession
Restoration
Symmetrical

1. _____ is the process of bringing back to a functional permanent unit.

2. _____ is the act or process of discovering decay.

3. The place where something divides into branches or separates (like roots on a tooth) is called a _____.

4. _____ is to have movement.

5. The branch of biology that deals with the form and structure of organisms without attention to function is

_____.

6. To touch or feel for abnormalities within soft tissue is _____.

7. _____ means outside the oral cavity.

8. The periodontal probe is used for

_____ and measuring the periodontal socket.

9. _____ is to recede or wear away from the normal location.

10. _____ is below the gingival tissue that surrounds a tooth.

11. An object is _____ when it is balanced on both sides.

12. _____ means within the oral cavity.

MULTIPLE CHOICE

Complete each question by circling the best answer.

1. The four reasons that a patient will see a dentist are:

   a. close to home, reasonable in price, pleasant décor, and nice dentist.
   b. as a new patient, in an emergency, for a consultation, and as a returning patient.
   c. sterile techniques, knowledgeable staff, appropriate attire, and clean environment.
   d. takes insurance, has flexible hours, performs specialty procedures, and no waiting.

2. What diagnostic techniques could be used to detect decay within a tooth?

   a. Visual evaluation
   b. Instrumentation
   c. Radiography
   d. All of the above

3. Which is not a color of tooth restorations?

   a. Silver
   b. Gold
   c. Platinum
   d. Tooth color

4. What charting symbols indicate a tooth that is not visible in the mouth?

   a. Circle around the tooth
   b. Outline with diagonal lines
   c. X through the tooth
   d. a and c

5. What is intraoral imaging similar to?

   a. Video camera
   b. Laser
   c. X-ray
   d. Photocopy

6. What classifications may involve premolars and molars?

   a. I
   b. II
   c. III
   d. a and b

7. What classifications involve incisors?

   a. I
   b. II
   c. III
   d. b and c

8. How would an MOD amalgam on tooth #4 be charted?

   a. The gingival third on the facial surface is outlined in blue and colored in
   b. The mesial, occlusal, and distal surface are outlined in blue and colored in
   c. The occlusal surface is outlined in blue with an *A* placed in the center
   d. The mesial and distal surfaces of the tooth are outlined in red and the occlusal portion is colored blue

9. What dental professional can perform the periodontal and screening recording on a patient?

   a. Dentist
   b. Assistant
   c. Hygienist
   d. a and c

10. What number exhibits extreme mobility?

    a. 0
    b. 1
    c. 2
    d. 3

CASE STUDY

Chart the following findings on the diagram:

#1	Impacted
#2	DO amalgam
#3	MOD amalgam
#4	Porcelain crown
#5–7	Three-unit gold bridge
#8	Root canal with a porcelain crown
#9	Root canal with a porcelain crown
#10	Class V composite
#11	Class V decay
#12	MO composite
#13	Abscess
#14	Class I lingual pit amalgam, with a sealant placed on the occlusal surface
#15	Sealant on occlusal surface
#16–17	Impacted
#18–21	Four-unit gold bridge, with 18 having a root canal
#24	Mesial composite
#25	Distal composite
#26	Fractured mesial/incisal edge
#28	MO composite
#29	Missing
#30	MOD amalgam decay
#31	O amalgam with recurrent decay
#32	Impacted

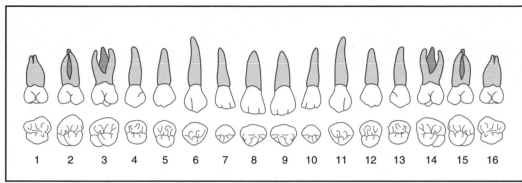

Right   Left

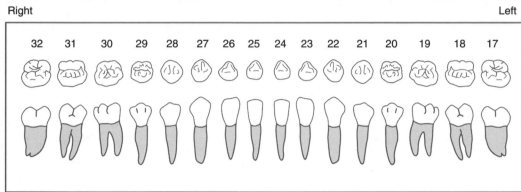

From your charting, answer the following questions:

1. What teeth do the bridges replace?
2. How many appointments will this patient require to complete his or her dental needs?
3. Is there an area within the mouth in which drifting could take place? If so, where would this occur?

4. Why do you think the dentist chose to place composite in teeth #12 and #28?
5. What teeth would be of concern for the oral and maxillofacial surgeon?

29 | The Medically and Physically Compromised Patient

SHORT ANSWER QUESTIONS

1. List the stages of the older population.
2. List the orally related conditions that affect older patients.
3. Describe the importance of the medical history for medically compromised patients.
4. List the major medical disorders that may affect the way a patient is treated in the dental office.
5. Describe the type of dental management a medically compromised patient would receive.

FILL IN THE BLANK

Select the best term from the list below and complete the following statements.

Aging
Alzheimer's
Anemia
Angina
Arthritis
Asthma
Atrophy
Aura
Bacteremia
Bronchitis
Cannula
Dementia
Diabetes
Emphysema
Endocarditis
Epilepsy
Hemophilia
Hyperplasia
Hyperthyroid
Hypothyroid
Infarction
Leukemia
Myocardial
Seizure
Stroke
Xerostomia

1. A deficiency in the oxygen-carrying component of the blood is a(n)

   _____.

2. A person who is diagnosed with

   _____ has a loss of memory, concentration, and judgment.

3. Wasting away or deterioration is called

   _____.

4. The sensation that precedes the onset of

   certain disorders is a(n) _____.

5. A(n) _____ is a sudden attack, spasm, or convulsion that occurs in specific disorders.

6. The presence of bacteria in the blood is

   termed _____.

7. _____ is the loss of saliva production that causes a dry mouth.

8. A medical condition that is known as a

   metabolic disorder is _____.

9. _____ is severe pain in the chest resulting from an insufficient supply of blood to the heart.

10. _____ is a condition of the lungs with an abnormal increase in the size of the air spaces, resulting in labored breathing and an increased susceptibility to infection.

11. _____ is the inflammation of the endocardium.

12. A neurological disorder with sudden recurring seizures of motor, sensory, or psychic malfunction is

    _____.

13. _____ refers to becoming mature or older.

14. _____ is a disease marked by progressive loss of mental range that results from degeneration of the brain cells.

15. A blood coagulation disorder in which the blood fails to clot normally is

    _____.

16. _____ is an abnormal increase in the number of cells in an organ or a tissue.

17. _____ is the inflammation of the mucous membrane of the bronchial tubes.

18. A flexible tube that is inserted into a bodily opening is a(n)

    _____.

19. _____ is a condition resulting from excessive activity of the thyroid gland.

20. _____ is an area of tissue that undergoes necrosis as a result of obstruction of blood supply in that area.

21. _____ is a disease of bone marrow in which there is abnormal development of white blood cells.

22. _____ is the muscular tissue of the heart.

23. Inflammation of a joint or many joints resulting in pain and swelling are

    symptoms of _____.

24. _____ is a chronic respiratory disease, often associated with allergies. It is characterized by sudden recurring attacks of labored breathing, chest constriction, and coughing.

25. _____ is a condition resulting from severe thyroid insufficiency.

26. Sudden loss of brain function caused by a blockage or rupture of a blood vessel to the brain is known as a(n)

    _____.

MULTIPLE CHOICE

Complete each question by circling the best answer.

1. What act protects people with special needs?
   a. State dental practice act
   b. Americans with Disabilities Act
   c. Good Samaritan Act
   d. Federal Food, Drug, and Cosmetic Act

2. What is the fastest-growing segment of the population?
   a. Infants
   b. Young adults
   c. Middle-aged adults
   d. Older adults

3. In which category would a 76-year-old patient fit?
   a. Young
   b. Young old
   c. Old
   d. Old old

4. Xerostomia is a condition of:
   a. excess saliva.
   b. eye infection.
   c. loss of hearing.
   d. dry mouth.

5. What oral health conditions affect the aging population?
   a. Periodontal disease
   b. Decay
   c. Bone resorption
   d. All of the above

6. Dementia is a condition of:

   a. bone loss.
   b. deterioration of metal capacity.
   c. aging.
   d. the body's senses.

7. What common side effect occurs from taking Dilantin?

   a. Hyperplasia
   b. Allergies
   c. Endocarditis
   d. Anxiety

8. What is another term for cerebrovascular accident?

   a. Angina
   b. Stroke
   c. Seizure
   d. Alzheimer's

9. An example of a neurological disorder is:

   a. emphysema.
   b. multiple sclerosis.
   c. Parkinson's disease.
   d. b and c

10. What is the leading cause of death in the United States?

    a. Emphysema
    b. Eating disorders
    c. Heart disease
    d. Drug abuse

11. What anesthetic agent is *not* recommended for patients with heart disease?

    a. Nitrous oxide/oxygen
    b. Epinephrine
    c. Carbocaine
    d. Novocain

12. Another term for hypertension is:

    a. high blood pressure.
    b. seizure.
    c. depression.
    d. anemia.

13. What organ in the body is affected by pulmonary disorders?

    a. Heart
    b. Brain
    c. Lungs
    d. Kidneys

14. What does the abbreviation *COPD* stand for?

    a. Common older population disorders
    b. Category of pulmonary diseases
    c. Cardiovascular patients in dentistry
    d. Chronic obstructive pulmonary disease

15. What disorder is associated with an overactive thyroid gland?

    a. Eating
    b. Endocrine
    c. Pulmonary
    d. Blood

16. How is a Type I diabetic classified?

    a. Child
    b. Adult
    c. Insulin dependent
    d. Non–insulin dependent

17. Obsessive fasting or starving oneself is a condition called:

    a. bulimia.
    b. schizophrenia.
    c. anorexia nervosa.
    d. substance abuse.

18. How is bulimia classified as a disorder?

    a. Endocrine
    b. Musculoskeletal
    c. Behavioral
    d. Psychological

CASE STUDY

Josh Allen is a 37-year-old patient of the practice and has been diagnosed with multiple sclerosis. His condition has deteriorated such that he is now uses a wheelchair. He has called the office today to schedule an appointment to have two teeth restored.

1. Do you think that a certain time of day would be better for the dental team to see Josh? If so, what would be the best time of day to schedule Josh for his appointment?
2. Are there any specific drugs that Josh may be taking that should be noted before treatment? If so, what would they be?
3. Your dental treatment area is not designed to treat patients in a wheelchair, so where should Josh be seen?
4. Describe specific techniques that help the patient move from a wheelchair to the dental chair.
5. Describe specific techniques that protect the person moving a patient from the wheelchair to the dental chair.

30 | Principles of Pharmacology

SHORT ANSWER QUESTIONS

1. Differentiate between a drug's chemical, generic, and trade names.
2. Describe the stages a drug goes through once it enters the body.
3. List each part of a prescription.
4. Describe how medications are administered.
5. Define the DEA and why drugs are categorized in five schedules of the Controlled Substance Act.
6. List the effects of drug use.
7. Describe the classifications of drugs prescribed and their effects.
8. Cite the factors that influence effects of a drug.
9. Describe the use of drug reference materials.

FILL IN THE BLANK

Select the best term from the list below and complete the following statements.

Absorption
Distribution
Dosage
Dose
Drug
Ethical
Excretion
Generic
Inscription
Metabolism
Patent
Pharmacology
Prescription
Prophylaxis
Signature
Subscription
Superscription
Systemic

1. _____ is the process of removing waste from blood, tissue, and organs.

2. _____ is the act of disbursement.

3. A person is _____ when they accept principles of right and wrong.

4. The _____ is the patient's name, address, date, and Rx on the prescription.

5. The term _____ relates to affecting a specific system of the body.

6. A specified quantity of a drug or medicine is termed a(n) _____.

7. _____ is a substance used in the diagnosis, treatment, or prevention of a disease.

8. The body goes through _____ when taking a drug.

9. A signed message is a(n) _____.

10. The body's _____ is a normal process that occurs to help in the maintenance of life.

11. The _____ are specific instructions on a prescription as how to take a specific medicine.

12. A(n) _____ is the amount of drug to be administered.

13. The official document or creation of a new drug will receive a(n) _____ before being marketed.

14. _____ is the science of drugs.

15. A(n) _____ is a written order to the pharmacist.

16. Patients may be prescribed a(n)

    _____ to protect them from getting a disease.

17. The _____ are the directions to the pharmacist for mixing the medication.

18. A(n) _____ product, such as a drug, is sold without a brand name or trademark.

MULTIPLE CHOICE

Complete each question by circling the best answer.

1. Where do drugs come from?

    a. Plants
    b. Animals
    c. Laboratory
    d. All of the above

2. What type of drug name is Advil?

    a. Generic name
    b. Brand name
    c. Chemical name
    d. Company name

3. The slowest route of absorption for a drug is:

    a. intramuscular.
    b. rectal.
    c. oral.
    d. intravenous.

4. Who is responsible for regulating the sale of medicines?

    a. Pharmaceutical companies
    b. Public health departments
    c. Centers for Disease Control
    d. Food and Drug Administration

5. Within the dental profession, who can prescribe drugs to a patient?

    a. Oral surgeon
    b. General dentist
    c. Dental hygienist
    d. a and b

6. What part of the prescription includes the name of the drug and quantity?

    a. Subscription
    b. Inscription
    c. Superscription
    d. Description

7. The abbreviation *b.i.d.* represents:

    a. once a day.
    b. twice a day.
    c. every 4 hours.
    d. take with food.

8. If a medication were placed sublingually, where would it be placed?

    a. Ancillary
    b. Rectally
    c. Under the tongue
    d. Topically

9. Where would a subcutaneous injection be given?

    a. Muscular
    b. Intravenous
    c. Nerve
    d. Under the skin

10. What schedule type would Tylenol with Codeine come under?

    a. I
    b. II
    c. III
    d. IV

11. When the body reacts to a drug, what does the person experience?

    a. Side effect
    b. Response
    c. Fever
    d. Hallucination

12. An analgesic would be prescribed for:

    a. hives.
    b. fever.
    c. relief of pain.
    d. b and c

13. Give an example of an antibiotic.

    a. Aspirin
    b. Codeine
    c. Erythromycin
    d. Meperidine

14. Which drug is prescribed to slow the clotting of blood?

    a. Aspirin
    b. Valium
    c. Coumadin
    d. Monistat

15. What type of drug may be prescribed for a patient with a cold?

    a. Dilantin
    b. Prozac
    c. Sudafed
    d. Ventolin

CASE STUDY

Mr. John Miller is scheduled to come in for periodontal surgery this morning. While setting up the treatment area for surgery, you remove the patient's radiographs and health history for the dentist's review. While assembling the documents, you notice an alert sticker indicating that Mr. Miller has a heart murmur and is allergic to penicillin.

1. What is an alert sticker?
2. Will Mr. Miller's heart murmur influence today's procedure? If so, how?
3. What should be considered when treating a patient with a heart murmur?
4. Why is it so important to know that Mr. Miller is allergic to penicillin?
5. Should a prescription been given to Mr. Miller prior to today's appointment? If so, when should Mr. Miller have taken the medicine?

31 | Assisting in a Medical Emergency

SHORT ANSWER QUESTIONS

1. Describe how to prevent a possible medical emergency.
2. List the appropriate qualifications that the dental assistant must have in emergency preparedness.
3. List the basic items that must be included in an emergency kit.
4. Discuss the use of a defibrillator during an emergency.
5. Describe the common signs and symptoms of an emergency and recognize them.
6. Define specific emergency situations and how to respond.

FILL IN THE BLANK

Select the best term from the list below and complete the following statements.

Acute
Airway
Allergen
Allergy
Anaphylaxis
Antibodies
Antigen
Aspiration
Asthma
Cardiopulmonary
Circulation
Convulsion
Erythema
Fibrillation
Gait
Hyperglycemia
Hypersensitivity
Hyperventilation
Hypoglycemia
Hypotension
Infarction
Myocardial
Physiological
Psychological
Resuscitation

Syncope
Unconsciousness
Ventricular

1. When a patient is _____, he or she is without control of his or her body.

2. _____ relates to the chambers of the heart.

3. A movement or passage of blood through vessels is the process of _____.

4. A(n)_____ is an involuntary muscular contraction.

5. _____ is a redness that is most likely caused by inflammation or infection.

6. _____ deals with mental processes and human behavior.

7. _____ is the means of restoring consciousness or life.

8. A rapid onset of a symptom is said to be _____.

9. The _____ is a passage through which air circulates.

10. A person who is highly sensitive to a certain substance is said to have an _____ to that substance.

11. A(n) _____ is a substance, such as pollen, that causes an allergy.

12. _____ is the loss of consciousness by a lack of blood going to the brain.

13. _____ is the rapid twitching of muscle fibers.

14. A person's _____ is his or her particular way or manner of moving by foot.

15. _____ is a chronic respiratory disease.

16. _____ involves both the heart and lungs.

17. _____ is sometimes a life-threatening hypersensitivity to a substance.

18. _____ are an immunoglobulin produced by lymphoid tissue in response to a foreign substance.

19. A substance that is introduced into the body to stimulate the production of an antibody is termed a(n) _____.

20. _____ is the act of inhaling something into the mouth.

21. An abnormally low level of glucose in the blood is the condition of _____.

22. _____ is abnormally low blood pressure.

23. A(n) _____ occurs when an area of heart tissue undergoes necrosis as a result of obstruction of blood supply.

24. The term for the muscular tissue of the heart is _____.

25. _____ is the complete functioning of the body.

26. An abnormally high presence of glucose in the blood is the condition of _____.

27. A person who is highly sensitive to a substance is said to be _____.

28. _____ is when a patient is breathing abnormally fast or deep.

MULTIPLE CHOICE

Complete each question by circling the best answer.

1. The best way to prevent an emergency is to:
   a. have the drug kit open and ready for all procedures.
   b. know your patient.
   c. call a patient's physician before his or her appointment.
   d. take vital signs in the reception area.

2. Most medical emergencies occur because people are:
   a. overweight.
   b. not taking their medication.
   c. under stress.
   d. not active.

3. Who is responsible for an individual's safety in the dental office?
   a. Dental assistant
   b. Dental hygienist
   c. Business assistant
   d. Dentist

4. Who in the dental office would most likely be in charge of calling the emergency medical services?
   a. Dentist
   b. Business assistant
   c. Dental laboratory technician
   d. Another patient

5. Where should emergency phone numbers be kept?

    a. Next to each phone
    b. In each treatment area
    c. In the business area
    d. In the sterilization area

6. What minimum credentials must a dental assistant have for emergency care standards?

    a. RN license
    b. CPR and Heimlich certification
    c. EMT certification
    d. DDS

7. In emergency care the abbreviation *abc* stands for:

    a. always be certified.
    b. absence of breathing and circulation.
    c. airway, breathing, and circulation.
    d. analyze before continuing.

8. What is the ratio of breaths to compressions for an adult victim when performing CPR?

    a. 1 breath / 5 compressions
    b. 2 breaths / 7 compressions
    c. 2 breaths / 15 compressions
    d. 3 breaths / 20 compressions

9. The most effective substance in a medical emergency is:

    a. an ammonia capsule.
    b. nitroglycerin.
    c. epinephrine.
    d. oxygen.

10. What does the abbreviation *AED* stand for?

    a. Automated external defibrillator
    b. Auxiliary examination device
    c. Acute emergency drill
    d. Airway that is externally directed

11. What is the danger of ventricular fibrillation?

    a. Electrocution
    b. Prevents the heart from pumping blood
    c. Increases the blood pressure
    d. Decreases the pulse rate

12. If a patient tells you how he or she feels, this is referred to as a:

    a. feeling.
    b. explanation.
    c. sign.
    d. symptom.

13. When a patient is unresponsive to sensory stimulation, he or she is said to be:

    a. unresponsive.
    b. unconscious.
    c. comatose.
    d. paralyzed.

14. What is the medical term for fainting?

    a. Stroke
    b. Seizure
    c. Syncope
    d. Senile

15. The medical term for chest pain is:

    a. angioplasty.
    b. angina.
    c. angiogram.
    d. anemia.

16. The medical term for a stroke is:

    a. cerebrovascular accident.
    b. cardiovascular accident.
    c. cardiopulmonary obstruction.
    d. obstructed airway.

17. What medication will patients with asthma most commonly have with them?

    a. Nitroglycerin
    b. Insulin
    c. Bronchodilator
    d. Analgesic

18. What kind of allergic response can be life threatening?

    a. Grand mal seizure
    b. Anaphylaxis
    c. Myocardial infarction
    d. Airway obstruction

19. An abnormal increase of glucose in the blood causes:

    a. angina.
    b. hypoglycemia.
    c. seizure.
    d. hyperglycemia.

CASE STUDY

Renee Miller is a 26-year-old woman who is in her third trimester of pregnancy. Renee is scheduled to have a root canal on tooth #12. Her health history and treatment record show no indication of adverse reactions to prior treatment. Renee is seated in the dental chair, and pretreatment instructions have been given. The procedure goes well, and you are repositioning the chair in an upright position while the dentist is discussing posttreatment. Renee comments that she feels faint.

1. Should Renee be having dental treatment while she is pregnant? If so, what is your reason?

2. Why might Renee be feeling faint?
3. What type of medical emergency is Renee experiencing?
4. How do you respond to this medical emergency?
5. Is there anything that could have prevented Renee from feeling this way?

32 | The Dental Office

SHORT ANSWER QUESTIONS

1. Describe the six areas of the dental environment in maintaining a professional office.
2. Discuss the important qualities of the reception area.
3. Describe the goals to achieve when designing the dental treatment area.
4. List the main clinical equipment needed for the treatment areas.
5. Discuss the basic function of the dental unit.

FILL IN THE BLANK

Select the best term from the list below and complete the following statements.

Condensation
Consultation
Operatory
Rheostat
Subsupine
Supine
Triturate
Upright

1. The _____ position is one in which the patient's head is below the heart; it is most commonly used in emergency situations.

2. To mechanically mix something is to

   _____.

3. A(n) _____ is a type of meeting to discuss a diagnosis or treatment.

4. _____ is the process by which a liquid is removed from vapor.

5. A patient who is in the _____ position is in a vertical position.

6. A room designed for dental treatment is a(n) _____.

7. The _____ is a foot-controlled device to operate machinery.

8. The _____ position is where the head, chest, and knees are at the same level.

MULTIPLE CHOICE

Complete each question by circling the best answer.

1. What is an ideal temperature for the reception area?

   a. 68°
   b. 72°
   c. 75°
   d. 78°

2. What type of flooring would best for the clinical area?

   a. Carpet
   b. Wood
   c. Vinyl
   d. Tile

3. What items are important to have in the reception area?

   a. Seating
   b. Lighting
   c. Reading material
   d. All of the above

4. Where does dental treatment take place in the dental office?

   a. Operatory
   b. Laboratory
   c. Business office
   d. Sterilization area

5. Another term for *operatory* is:

   a. rheostat.
   b. treatment area.
   c. radiography.
   d. laboratory.

6. In which chair position are most dental procedures completed?

    a. Upright
    b. Subsupine
    c. Supine
    d. Flat

7. Which two items are found on the dental assistant's stool that are not seen on the operator's stool?

    a. Light switch and up-and-down button
    b. Back cushion and wheeled coasters
    c. Headrest and armrests
    d. Footrest and abdominal bar

8. What foot-controlled device is used to operate the dental handpieces?

    a. Dental unit
    b. Amalgamator
    c. Rheostat
    d. Central air compressor

9. What does the abbreviation *HVE* stand for?

    a. High-volume evacuator
    b. Hose vacuum
    c. Hold vacuum evacuator
    d. Handle volume evacuator

10. Where do you place dental materials to be triturated?

    a. Dental unit
    b. Amalgamator
    c. Rheostat
    d. Central air compressor

CASE STUDY

Imagine that you are responsible for introducing Nancy Drake to your dental practice. Nancy is the newly hired dental assistant. She has been in dentistry for 26 years and is quite familiar with her role as a professional. She has mentioned that she really likes the design and setup of the dental office, and is excited about adding her personal touches to make the office more functional.

1. What would be your role in showing Nancy the office and how it is set up?
2. The office has four dental treatment areas, and three full-time dental assistants. How can each assistant create an environment in which he or she feels comfortable?
3. What kinds of personal items can be brought in to give the dental office more of a team atmosphere?

33 | Delivering Dental Care

SHORT ANSWER QUESTIONS

1. Describe how you would prepare for patient arrival.
2. Discuss the importance in preparing a dental treatment room for patient treatment.
3. Describe how the operator is positioned during treatment.
4. Describe how the assistant is positioned during treatment.
5. Explain the instrument transfer technique.
6. Specify three grasps used by the operator.
7. Identify five areas in which the assistant must be competent when practicing expanded functions.

FILL IN THE BLANK

Select the best term from the list below and complete the following statements.

Delegate
Direct supervision
Expanded function
Fulcrum
Grasp
Indirect supervision
Indirect vision

1. The dentist provides _____ by being within the same treatment area when overseeing someone's work.

2. _____ is used to view something through the use of a mirror.

3. A(n) _____ is a dental function that is delegated to someone by the dentist.

4. A(n) _____ becomes a finger rest when holding an instrument or handpiece.

5. A(n) _____ is used to hold a specific instrument or handpiece.

6. The dentist provides _____ by being in the immediate area when overseeing someone's work.

7. To _____ is to comment or entrust a specific assignment to another person.

MULTIPLE CHOICE

Complete each question by circling the best answer.

1. What can increase productivity in the dental office?

   a. Increase patient comfort
   b. Minimize stress and fatigue
   c. Practice expanded functions
   d. All of the above

2. When using the clock concept, where is the static zone located?

   a. 12:00 to 2:00
   b. 2:00 to 4:00
   c. 4:00 to 7:00
   d. 7:00 to 12:00

3. Using the clock concept, where are instruments exchanged during a procedure?

   a. Static zone
   b. Assistant's zone
   c. Transfer zone
   d. Operator zone

4. Besides the assistant, what is located in the assistant's zone?

   a. Dental unit
   b. Mobile cabinet
   c. Assistant stool
   d. b and c

5. In relation to the operator, how should the assistant be positioned?

   a. Same height
   b. Higher than the operator
   c. Level with the patient's head
   d. Lower than the operator

6. How should the operator maintain his or her posture when treating a patient?

    a. Upright
    b. Elbows at his or her side
    c. Feet flat on the ground
    d. All of the above

7. The assistant should use _____ hand(s) in instrument transfer.

    a. both
    b. one
    c. varying

8. What hand is used primarily to transfer instruments to a right-handed dentist?

    a. Left
    b. Right
    c. Either

9. Indirect vision is accomplished with a:

    a. light.
    b. mouth mirror.
    c. explorer.
    d. glasses.

10. Another term for finger rest is:

    a. rheostat.
    b. intraoral.
    c. fulcrum.
    d. tactile.

CASE STUDY

Dr. Williams is a general dentist who has been practicing dentistry for 35 years. He views his dental assistants and dental hygienists as an important part of the practice and recognizes everyone as a contributor to patient care. Dr. Williams is an advocate of advanced functions and feels that dental assistants should be allowed to practice procedures that are legal.

1. How can you find out what procedures are legal for you to practice in your state?
2. As you begin your clinical training, describe specific skills that you could practice to help become more proficient in expanded functions.
3. What ways can you maintain a high level of competency when performing advanced functions?
4. If there were a new clinical procedure that became an advanced function in your state, how would you acquire the knowledge and skill to practice it?
5. Are there any procedures that you feel a dental assistant could perform that are not legal at this time?

34 | Dental Hand Instruments

SHORT ANSWER QUESTIONS

1. Describe the three parts of a dental hand instrument.
2. Describe the instrument formula designed by G.V. Black.
3. List the examination instruments and their use.
4. List the types of hand-cutting instruments and their use.
5. List the types of restorative instruments and their use.
6. Describe additional accessory instruments used in dentistry.
7. Describe the use of preset trays and tubs in dentistry.
8. Discuss the theory of placing instruments in a specific sequence.

FILL IN THE BLANK

Select the best term from the list below and complete the following statements.

Beveled
Blade
Handle
Nib
Plane
Point
Serrated
Shank
Tactile
Working end

1. _____ means to have a sense of touch or feeling.

2. The _____ is the portion of a dental instrument that is used on the tooth or for mixing dental materials.

3. The portion of a dental instrument that the operator grasps is the _____.

4. The working end of an instrument can be _____, or at an angle.

5. A flat edge of the working end of an instrument that is sharp enough to cut is called a _____.

6. A sharp point or tip is called the _____.

7. An instrument that is _____ has notchlike projections extending from a flat surface.

8. A flat or level surface is the _____.

9. The _____ is the portion of a dental instrument that attaches the handle to the working end.

10. A _____ can be a sharp or tapered end.

MULTIPLE CHOICE

Complete each question by circling the best answer.

1. What dental instruments are more commonly referred to by a number than by a name?

   a. Mirrors
   b. Restorative
   c. Pliers
   d. Excavators

2. What part of the instrument is located between the handle and the working end?

   a. Nib
   b. Shank
   c. Blade
   d. Plane

3. What classification of instruments is used to manually remove decay?

   a. Examination
   b. Hand-cutting
   c. Restorative
   d. Accessory

4. Besides indirect vision, what can the mouth mirror be used for?

   a. Moisture control
   b. Anesthesia procedure
   c. Retraction
   d. Charting of teeth

5. The main characteristic of the working end of an explorer is:

   a. dull.
   b. flat.
   c. serrated.
   d. pointed.

6. What instrument is part of the basic setup?

   a. Spoon excavator
   b. Cotton pliers
   c. Condenser
   d. Carver

7. What instrument is used to measure the sulcus of a tooth?

   a. Spoon excavator
   b. Cotton pliers
   c. Explorer
   d. Periodontal probe

8. What instrument is similar to the spoon excavator in appearance and use?

   a. Explorer
   b. Black spoon
   c. Discoid-cleoid
   d. Gingival margin trimmer

9. What instrument would be used to carve the interproximal portion of an amalgam restoration?

   a. Black spoon
   b. Discoid-cleoid
   c. Gingival margin trimmer
   d. Hollenback

10. What instrument is used to pack down amalgam?

    a. Cotton pliers
    b. Amalgam knife
    c. Condenser
    d. Burnisher

11. What kind of instrument is a discoid-cleoid?

    a. Carver
    b. Examination
    c. Hand-cutting
    d. Packing

12. What type of scissors would be placed on a restorative tray setup?

    a. Tissue
    b. Suture
    c. Crown and bridge
    d. Surgical

13. Howe pliers are also referred to as:

    a. cotton pliers.
    b. 110.
    c. articulating.
    d. chisel.

14. The newly mixed amalgam is placed in the

    _____ before transferring it in the amalgam carrier.

    a. syringe
    b. cotton pliers
    c. spoon excavator
    d. amalgam well

CASE STUDY

You are assisting in a class II amalgam procedure on tooth #29. In order of use, list the instruments that would be in the setup, beginning from the left and working toward the right of the tray. Under each instrument, describe the use of that instrument for this procedure.

35 | Dental Handpieces and Accessories

SHORT ANSWER QUESTIONS

1. Discuss the historical importance of the dental handpiece.
2. Describe the low-speed handpiece and its use in dentistry.
3. Describe the attachments used on the low-speed handpiece.
4. Describe the high-speed handpiece and its use.
5. Give a brief description of other types of handpieces used in dentistry.
6. Describe rotary instruments and how they are used.
7. List the parts of a bur.
8. Give the composition, shape, and use of the carbide and diamond burs.

FILL IN THE BLANK

Select the best term from the list below and complete the following statements.

Console
Flutes
Mandrel
Rotary
Shank
Ultrasonic

1. A(n) _____ instrument is a part or device that rotates around an axis.

2. The _____ or grooves in the cutting portion of a bur resemble pleats.

3. A(n) _____ is a freestanding cabinet to hold something.

4. The narrow portion of the bur that fits into the handpiece is called a(n)

   _____.

5. A(n) _____ device converts sound waves into mechanical energy.

6. Sandpaper discs are mounted on a(n)

   _____, which is a metal shaft in which a working tool is mounted on.

MULTIPLE CHOICE

Complete each question by circling the best answer.

1. How did the first handpiece operate?

   a. Foot pedal
   b. Electric
   c. Belt driven
   d. Water

2. What are the two most common handpieces used in dentistry?

   a. Low-speed
   b. High-speed
   c. Contra-angle
   d. a and b

3. How fast can the low-speed handpiece go?

   a. 10,000 rpm
   b. 20,000 rpm
   c. 30,000 rpm
   d. 40,000 rpm

4. What attachment is used to hold the bristle brush and prophy cup?

   a. Prophy angle
   b. Contra-angle
   c. High-speed
   d. Mandrel

5. How fast can the high-speed handpiece rotate?

   a. 250,000 rpm
   b. 450,000 rpm
   c. 650,000 rpm
   d. 950,000 rpm

6. How is a tooth kept cool and clean during the use of the high-speed handpiece?

   a. Air
   b. Suction system
   c. Water coolant
   d. Application of a dental material

7. How does the high-speed handpiece hold a bur?

   a. Friction grip
   b. Locking key
   c. Latch type
   d. Twist and lock

8. On the high-speed handpiece, the

   _____ light
   helps illuminate the working field.

   a. water
   b. air
   c. fiber-optic
   d. suction

9. What type of handpiece resembles a sandblaster?

   a. Laser
   b. Low-speed
   c. Air abrasion
   d. High-speed

10. A(n) _____ shank fits into the contra-angle attachment.

    a. friction grip
    b. mandrel
    c. long
    d. latch type

11. Restorative burs are made from what material?

    a. Stainless steel
    b. Tungsten carbide
    c. Gold
    d. Nickel

12. What design of bur is a 331/2?

    a. Round
    b. Tapered
    c. Inverted cone
    d. Pear

13. The advantage of using a diamond bur is its:

    a. cutting ability.
    b. fineness.
    c. polishing ability.
    d. nonabrasiveness.

14. Finishing burs are used on what type of dental material?

    a. Amalgam
    b. Porcelain
    c. Gold
    d. Composites

15. What is used to hold a disc in the handpiece?

    a. Contra-angle attachment
    b. Bur
    c. Mandrel
    d. Prophy angle

CASE STUDY

Your tray setup for the next patient in the treatment area includes a high-speed handpiece, low-speed motor, contra-angle attachment, #169 friction grip bur, and a #4 round latch-type bur.

1. How do you know which hose on the dental unit to attach to the high-speed handpiece?
2. To which handpiece do you attach the contra-angle attachment?
3. On which handpiece do you insert the #169 bur?
4. On which handpiece do you insert the #4 round bur?

36 | Moisture Control

SHORT ANSWER QUESTIONS

1. List the isolation techniques used to decrease moisture during a dental procedure.
2. Give the two types of oral evacuation systems used in dentistry.
3. Describe the grasp and positioning of the high-volume oral evacuator tip.
4. Give the use of the air-water syringe.
5. Describe the dental dam and its role in moisture control.
6. List the equipment and supplies for dental dam application.
7. Describe special situations in the preparation and placement of the dental dam.

FILL IN THE BLANK

Select the best term from the list below and complete the following statements.

Beveled
Bow
Exposed
Invert
Isolated
Jaw
Malaligned
Septum
Stylus
Universal

1. When an item is separated from others like it, it is said to be _____.

2. _____ are two opposing hinges that pull apart from each other.

3. A(n) _____ surface is one angle of a surface that meets another angle.

4. To turn inside out is to

_____.

5. A bend or curve downward is termed a(n) _____.

6. The rubber dam punch has a(n)

_____, which is a sharp-pointed tool used for cutting.

7. An instrument or item that is adaptable or adjustable to many sizes is said to be

_____.

8. When an object is not in a straight row it is _____.

9. A(n) _____ is a thin membrane that separates two items.

10. When an object is made visible, it becomes _____.

MULTIPLE CHOICE

Complete each question by circling the best answer.

1. What are the two types of evacuators used in dental procedures?

   a. Cotton rolls and saliva ejector
   b. High-volume suction, saliva ejector
   c. Dental dam and high-volume suction
   d. Air-water syringe and saliva ejector

2. The main function of the saliva ejector is to:

   a. remove dental materials.
   b. remove blood.
   c. remove saliva and water.
   d. remove tooth fragments.

3. What type of materials are operative suction tips made from?

   a. Glass
   b. Metal
   c. Plastic
   d. b and c

4. What type of rinsing technique is completed during a procedure?

   a. Limited
   b. Full
   c. Gargle
   d. Spray

5. What methods of isolation are most commonly used in a dental procedure?

   a. Dental dam
   b. Cotton rolls
   c. Gauze
   d. a and b

6. What type of isolation would commonly be chosen for shorter procedures?

   a. Dental dam
   b. Cotton rolls
   c. Gauze squares
   d. Saliva ejector

7. Why is it important to wet a cotton roll before removal?

   a. Can interfere with the dental materials setting
   b. Can stick to the teeth
   c. Can pull on the mucosa
   d. Can be sucked up in the suction tip

8. Teeth that are visible through the dam are referred to as being:

   a. open.
   b. exposed.
   c. revealed.
   d. decayed.

9. What piece of equipment stabilizes and stretches the dam away from the tooth?

   a. Dental dam frame
   b. Dental dam clamp
   c. Ligature tie
   d. Dental dam forceps

10. If you are unable to slide the dam interproximally, what could be placed on the underside of the dam to help in the application?

    a. Water
    b. Vaseline
    c. Water-soluble lubricant
    d. Powder

11. What hole size on the rubber dam punch is the smallest size?

    a. 0
    b. 1
    c. 3
    d. 6

12. When would you use an anterior dental dam clamp?

    a. Class I
    b. Class II
    c. Class V
    d. Class VI

CASE STUDY

Candy Allen is having a Class III composite resin placed on tooth #8 today. Candy has had many restorations placed and is very comfortable with the dental treatment she receives. Throughout the procedure it will be your responsibility to provide moisture control.

1. Following the administration of anesthesia, what type of moisture control would be used?
2. The dentist has asked you to place the dental dam. At what point of the procedure will you place the dental dam?
3. What teeth should be isolated?
4. How will the dental dam be held in place?
5. When will the dental dam be removed in this procedure?

37 | Anesthesia and Pain Control in Dentistry

SHORT ANSWER QUESTIONS

1. Discuss the importance of pain control in dentistry.
2. Describe the chemical makeup and application of topical anesthetic.
3. Discuss the chemical makeup and application of local anesthetic agents.
4. Describe nitrous oxide–oxygen sedation and why it is used in dentistry.
5. Discuss the importance in reducing the exposure of the dental team to nitrous oxide–oxygen.
6. Discuss intravenous sedation and how it is used in dentistry.
7. Discuss general anesthesia and how it is used in dentistry.

FILL IN THE BLANK

Select the best term from the list below and complete the following statements.

Analgesia
Diffuse
Duration
Gauge
Innervation
Lumen
Oximetry
Permeated
Porous
Systemic
Tidal volume
Titrate
Toxicity
Vasoconstrictor

1. _____ is the quality or condition of something that may be harmful to the body.

2. _____ relates to affecting a specific system within the body, or affecting the entire system.

3. The amount of air inhaled and exhaled at each breath is the _____.

4. Anesthesia will last a(n) _____ or a period of time.

5. A standard dimension or measurement is a _____.

6. A(n) _____ is an inner open space.

7. _____ is the means to measure oxygen in the blood.

8. _____ produces numbing or absence of sense of pain.

9. A(n) _____ is the constriction of a blood vessel either by a nerve or by a drug.

10. To spread out or scatter is to _____.

11. To determine the concentration of a substance you would _____ it.

12. An item that is _____ allows a substance to spread or flow throughout.

13. Something that is _____ will have openings to allow gas or fluid to pass through.

14. The _____ of nerves spreads into and supplies an organ or body part.

MULTIPLE CHOICE

Complete each question by circling the best answer.

1. Why are topical anesthetics used in dentistry?

    a. To sedate the patient
    b. To numb the localized nerves
    c. To numb the surface tissue
    d. For inhalation sedation

2. What is the most frequently selected form of pain control used in dentistry?

    a. Prescribed drugs
    b. Local anesthesia
    c. Nitrous oxide–oxygen sedation
    d. Intravenous sedation

3. Local anesthetics are injected near the

    _____ to create the numbing effect.

    a. artery
    b. vein
    c. nerve
    d. pulp

4. What can be added to a local anesthetic to prolong its effect?

    a. Alcohol
    b. Ammonia
    c. Nitrous
    d. Epinephrine

5. What injection technique do dentists most frequently use on maxillary teeth?

    a. Block
    b. Infiltration
    c. Intraosseous
    d. Intravenous

6. What needle sizes are most commonly used in dentistry?

    a. ½″ and ¾″
    b. 1″ and 2″
    c. 1½″ and 1″
    d. 1″ and 1″

7. Will a patient with an abscess get numb?

    a. No
    b. Only with anesthesia with a vasoconstrictor
    c. Yes
    d. Only on the maxillary

8. Paresthesia is what type of condition?

    a. Localized toxic reaction
    b. Injection into a blood vessel
    c. Numbness
    d. Infected area

9. What dentist first used nitrous oxide on his patients?

    a. G.V. Black
    b. Horace Wells
    c. C. Edmund Kells
    d. Pierre Fauchard

10. How can the dental team be at risk for exposure to nitrous oxide–oxygen?

    a. Leakage from the nasal mask
    b. Exhalation
    c. Leakage from the hoses
    d. All of the above

11. What is given at the beginning and end of a procedure when a patient receives nitrous oxide–oxygen?

    a. Local anesthesia
    b. Oxygen
    c. Gauze to bite down on
    d. Topical fluoride

12. What stage is a patient if he or she is conscious during IV sedation?

    a. Analgesia
    b. Excitement
    c. General anesthesia
    d. Respiratory failure

13. What level of anesthesia is a patient at during general anesthesia?

    a. Stage 1
    b. Stage 2
    c. Stage 3
    d. Stage 4

14. In what environment is general anesthesia most often given to dental patients?

    a. Dental office
    b. Outpatient clinic
    c. Hospital
    d. b and c

CASE STUDY

Meredith Smith is coming in today for a new bridge on teeth #3–5. She is apprehensive about what will be completed by the dentist. Ms. Smith has discussed the option of having nitrous oxide anesthesia during the procedure, and she seems reassured that this will help alleviate her worries.

1. What methods of anesthesia will most likely be provided for Ms. Smith today?

2. Could there be any contraindications that might prevent Ms. Smith from receiving any of the anesthesia methods that were mentioned? If so, give some examples.
3. Where would you find these contraindications?

4. What anesthesia would be given first to Ms. Smith?
5. What will be placed on the tray setup for this anesthesia procedure?

38 | Introduction to Oral Radiography

SHORT ANSWER QUESTIONS

1. Describe the uses of dental radiographs.
2. Describe the discovery of x-radiation.
3. Describe the process of ionization.
4. Describe the properties of x-radiation.
5. Describe in detail how x-rays are produced.
6. Label the parts of the dental x-ray tubehead and the dental x-ray tube.
7. Describe the effect of the kilovoltage on the quality of the x-ray beam.
8. Describe how milliamperage affects the quality of the x-ray beam.
9. Give the range of kilovoltage and milliamperage required for dental radiography.
10. Discuss the effects of radiation exposure on the human body.
11. Discuss the risks versus benefit of dental radiographs.
12. List critical organs that are sensitive to radiation.
13. Discuss the ALARA concept.
14. Describe methods of protecting the patient from excess radiation.
15. Describe methods of protecting the operator from excess radiation.

FILL IN THE BLANK

Select the best term from the list below and complete the following statements.

ALARA
Anode
Cathode
Contrast
Density
Dental radiography
Dose
Electron
Energy
Genetic effects
Ion
Ionizing radiation
Kilovoltage
Latent period
Milliampere
Peak
Penumbra matter
Photon
Primary beam
Radiation
Radiograph
Radiology
Somatic effects
Tungsten target
X-radiation
X-ray

1. _____ is the emission of energy in the forms of waves through space or through a material.

2. _____ is a high-energy ionizing electromagnetic radiation.

3. A form of ionizing radiation is the _____.

4. _____ is the science or study of radiation as used in medicine.

5. A(n) _____ is an image produced on photosensitive film by exposing the film to x-rays and then processing it.

6. The making of radiographs of the teeth and adjacent structures by exposure to x-rays is _____.

7. _____ is radiation that produces ionization.

8. The positive electrode in the x-ray tube is the _____.

9. The negative electrode in the x-ray tube is the _____.

10. The _____ is the most penetrating beam produced at the target of the anode.

11. An electrically charged particle is a(n) _____.

12. The _____ is the x-ray tube peak voltage used during an x-ray exposure.

13. _____ is 1/1000 of an ampere, a unit of measurement used to describe the intensity of an electric current.

14. A tiny, negatively charged particle found in the atom is a(n) _____.

15. The _____ is a focal spot in the anode.

16. _____ is the differences in degrees of blackness on a radiograph.

17. _____ is the overall darkness or blackness of a radiograph.

18. The amount of energy absorbed by tissues is its _____.

19. _____ are effects of radiation that are passed on to future generations through genetic cells.

20. Radiation that causes illness that is responsible for poor health is _____.

21. The period of time between exposure to ionizing radiation and the appearance of symptoms is the _____.

22. _____ is a concept of radiation protection that states all exposures should be kept "as low as reasonably achievable."

23. A _____ is a minute bundle of pure energy that has no weight or mass.

24. Anything that occupies space and has form or shape is _____.

25. The ability to do work takes _____.

26. The blurred or indistinct area that surrounds an image is _____.

MULTIPLE CHOICE

Complete each question by circling the best answer.

1. Who discovered x-rays?
   a. G.V. Black
   b. W.C. Roentgen
   c. Pierre Fauchard
   d. Horace Wells

2. Who was the first person to make practical use of radiographs in dentistry?
   a. C. Edmund Kells
   b. G.V. Black
   c. W.C. Roentgen
   d. Horace Wells

3. What is the process by which electrons are removed from electrically stable atoms?
   a. Physics
   b. Radiation
   c. Ionization
   d. Roentgen

4. The primary component of a dental x-ray machine is the:
   a. tubehead.
   b. PID.
   c. extension arm.
   d. all of the above

5. The name of the negative electrode inside the x-ray tube is the:
   a. cathode.
   b. nucleus.
   c. anode.
   d. photon.

6. The name of the positive electrode inside the x-ray tube is the:

   a. cathode.
   b. nucleus.
   c. anode.
   d. neutron.

7. What is located on the x-ray machine control panel?

   a. Filter
   b. Collimator
   c. Milliamperage (mA) selector
   d. Tubehead

8. During the production of x-rays, how much energy is lost as heat?

   a. 5%
   b. 25%
   c. 50%
   d. 99%

9. What are the types of radiation?

   a. Primary
   b. Secondary
   c. Scatter
   d. All of the above

10. A structure that appears dark on a processed radiograph is called:

    a. radiopaque.
    b. radiolucent.
    c. contrast.
    d. density.

11. A structure that appears light on a processed radiograph is called:

    a. radiopaque.
    b. density.
    c. contrast.
    d. radiolucent.

12. What exposure factor controls contrast?

    a. mA
    b. kVp
    c. Time
    d. Distance

13. Density is the:

    a. overall lightness of a processed radiograph.
    b. structure that appears light on a processed radiograph.
    c. overall darkness of a processed radiograph.
    d. structure that appears dark on a processed radiograph.

14. The harmful effects of x-rays are called:

    a. radiation.
    b. ionization.
    c. ultraviolet rays.
    d. infrared rays.

15. The period of time between x-ray exposure and appearance of symptoms is the:

    a. exposure time.
    b. primary radiation.
    c. development.
    d. latent period.

16. Radiation that is passed on to future generations has:

    a. cumulative effects.
    b. somatic effects.
    c. genetic effects.
    d. exposure effects.

17. A system used to measure radiation is the:

    a. traditional, or standard, system.
    b. metric system.
    c. Système Internationale.
    d. a and c

18. The maximum permissible dose of radiation for occupationally exposed persons is:

    a. 5.0 rem per year.
    b. 15 rem per year.
    c. 50 rem per year.
    d. .05 rem per year.

19. The purpose of the collimator is to:

    a. filter the primary beam.
    b. reduce the exposure of the primary beam.
    c. restrict the size of the primary beam.
    d. filter scatter radiation.

20. The purpose of the aluminum filter is to:

    a. reduce the exposure of the primary beam.
    b. remove low-energy, long-wavelength rays.
    c. restrict the size of the primary beam.
    d. remove high-energy, short-wavelength rays.

21. Which patients should wear a lead apron and thyroid collar?

    a. Patients with a pacemaker
    b. Patients with lung cancer
    c. Children
    d. All patients

22. The fastest film speed available today is:

    a. A-speed.
    b. F-speed.
    c. B-speed.
    d. C-speed.

23. The purpose of personnel monitoring is to:

    a. record the amount of radiation a patient receives.
    b. determine the amount of radiation exposing a radiograph.
    c. record the amount of radiation that reaches the body.
    d. check for radiation leakage.

24. What is the purpose of equipment monitoring?

    a. To record the amount of radiation a patient receives
    b. To determine the amount of radiation exposing a radiograph
    c. To record the amount of radiation that reaches the body
    d. To check for radiation leakage

25. What states that "all exposure to radiation should be kept to a minimum" or "as low as reasonably achievable"?

    a. The right-to-know law
    b. The ALARA concept
    c. Patients' bill of rights
    d. Dental creed

CASE STUDY

Your next patient is a 37-year-old woman who is new to the practice. She is scheduled today to have a series of x-rays taken. In reviewing the patient record, you notice that this patient has been diagnosed with leukemia and is currently receiving medical care.

1. Where in the patient record would you find this information about a patient?
2. What critical organ of the body is affected by leukemia?
3. What degree of sensitivity affects the cells or tissue of this organ?
4. It is obvious that this patient got the go-ahead to have x-rays taken. Who should be consulted about dental care when a person's health is questionable?
5. Why is it important to continue with a patient's dental care when he or she is medically compromised?

39 | Dental Film and Processing Radiographs

SHORT ANSWER QUESTIONS

1. Identify the types of dental x-ray film holders and devices.
2. Describe the composition of a dental x-ray film.
3. Describe the care and maintenance of the processing solutions, equipment, and equipment accessories used in manual and automatic film processing.
4. List and identify the component parts of an automatic film processor.
5. Describe the film processing problems that result from time and temperature errors.
6. Describe the film processing problems that result from chemical contamination.
7. Describe the film processing problems that result from film handling errors.
8. Describe the film processing problems that result from lighting errors.
9. State the types and indications for the three types of dental radiographs.
10. Identify the five basic sizes of intraoral dental x-ray film.
11. Explain the purpose of an intensifying screen.
12. Describe the process for duplicating radiographs.
13. Discuss the requirements necessary for the darkroom.

FILL IN THE BLANK

Select the best term from the list below and complete the following statements.

Automatic processing
Beam alignment devices
Bite-wing radiograph
Duplicating film
Extraoral film
Film cassette
Film emulsion
Film-holding devices
Film speed
Intensifying screen
Intraoral film

Label side
Latent image
Manual processing
Occlusal radiograph
Periapical radiograph
Processing errors
Tube side

1. A(n) _____ is the invisible image on the film after exposure but before processing.

2. A layer on the x-ray film that contains the x-ray sensitive crystals is the

   _____.

3. The _____ is the solid white side of the film that faces the x-ray tube.

4. The _____ is the colored side of the film that faces the tongue.

5. _____ is a method of film processing that uses film racks and processing tanks.

6. _____ is the automated method of film processing.

7. _____ are used to hold the film in position in the patient's mouth.

8. _____ are used to indicate the PID position in relation to the tooth and film.

9. _____ is film that is used for placement in the patient's mouth.

10. Film designed for use in cassettes is

    _____.

11. Film designed for use in film duplicating

    machines is _____.

12. A radiograph that shows the crown, root tip, and surrounding structures is

    a _____.

13. A(n) _____ shows the crowns of both arches on one film.

14. A radiograph that shows large areas of the maxilla or mandible is the

    _____.

15. The holder for extraoral films during

    exposure is a _____.

16. _____ is determined by the sensitivity of the emulsion on the film to radiation.

17. The _____ is used to convert x-ray energy into visible light, which in turn exposes screen film.

18. _____ are faults that occurred on the radiograph during processing.

MULTIPLE CHOICE

Complete each question by circling the best answer.

1. How does the use of film holders protect the patient from unnecessary radiation?

   a. Filters the scatter radiation
   b. Keeps the patient's hands and fingers from being exposed to x-radiation
   c. Speeds up the process
   d. Shows the correct teeth

2. Describe a basic type of film holder.

   a. Hemostat device
   b. Resembles a clothespin
   c. Square with adhesive on the back
   d. Bite-block with backing plate and slot for film retention

3. Name a component of an intraoral film.

   a. Film emulsion
   b. Aluminum foil
   c. Plastic
   d. Alginate

4. The image on the film before it is processed is the:

   a. density.
   b. latent image.
   c. contrast.
   d. mirror image.

5. Which side of the film faces toward the tube?

   a. Envelope-looking side
   b. Silver side
   c. Plain side
   d. Shiny side

6. What size film is used for periapical radiographs?

   a. 0
   b. 1
   c. 2
   d. 3

7. What size film is used for occlusal radiographs?

   a. 2
   b. 3
   c. 4
   d. 5

8. Describe the appearance of an extraoral film cassette.

   a. Flexible
   b. Rigid
   c. Expandable
   d. a and b

9. What converts x-ray energy into visible light?

   a. Aluminum foil
   b. Cardboard
   c. Intensifying screen
   d. Collimator

10. When would you need to duplicate a radiograph?

    a. For a second opinion
    b. Send to an insurance company
    c. Referring a patient to a specialist
    d. b and c

11. How should x-ray film be stored?

    a. Away from light
    b. In heat
    c. In a moist environment
    d. Submersed in chemicals

12. Where is the expiration date on a package of x-ray film?

    a. On each film
    b. Outside of the box
    c. On package insert
    d. In the bar code

13. What is the second step in processing dental radiographs?

    a. Developing
    b. Fixing
    c. Rinsing
    d. Washing

14. Which is the most popular form of processing solutions?

    a. Powdered
    b. Liquid concentrate
    c. Diluted
    d. Premixed

15. How often should processing solutions be replenished?

    a. Daily
    b. Weekly
    c. Bimonthly
    d. Monthly

16. What is a low-intensity light composed of long wavelengths in the red-orange spectrum?

    a. X-ray
    b. Safelight
    c. Intensifying screen
    d. Filter

17. What is the minimum distance between a safelight and the working area?

    a. 1 foot
    b. 2 feet
    c. 3 feet
    d. 4 feet

18. What is the optimum temperature for the water in the manual processing tanks?

    a. 65°
    b. 68°
    c. 72°
    d. 75°

19. What is the major advantage of automatic film processing?

    a. Better film
    b. Saves time
    c. Less chemicals
    d. Safer

20. Are manual processing solutions and automatic processing solutions interchangeable?

    a. Yes
    b. No

CASE STUDY

You are scheduled to take radiographs on the following patients. Listed below are the areas of the mouth where you will be taking the films. For each area, give the size of film that you will need to set up for the procedure.

1. Patient 1, a 28-year-old

Maxillary right molar:	Maxillary left molar:
Maxillary centrals:	Mandibular centrals:
Mandibular right molar:	Mandibular left molar:
Right bite-wing:	
Left bite-wing:	

2. Patient 2, an 8-year-old

Maxillary right molar:	Maxillary left molar:
Mandibular right molar:	Mandibular left molar:
Right bite-wing:	
Left bite-wing:	

3. Patient 3, a 4-year-old

   Maxillary occlusal:
   Mandibular occlusal:

40 | Legal Issues, Quality Assurance, and Infection Control in Radiography

SHORT ANSWER QUESTIONS

1. Describe informed consent with regard to dental radiographs.
2. Describe the types of laws affecting the practice of dental radiography.
3. Describe what is included in the Consumer-Patient Radiation Health and Safety Act.
4. Identify the individual who owns the dental radiographs.
5. Describe the purpose of a quality assurance program.
6. Describe the components of a quality assurance program.
7. Describe quality control tests for processing solutions.
8. Explain the use of a stepwedge.
9. Explain the purpose of a reference radiograph.
10. Explain the infection control requirements for preparing a radiography operatory.

FILL IN THE BLANK

Select the best term from the list below and complete the following statements.

Disclosure
Informed consent
Liable
Quality assurance
Quality control tests

1. _____ is the process of informing the patient about radiographic procedures.

2. _____ is permission granted by a patient after he or she has been informed about the particulars of the procedure.

3. _____ means that a person is accountable, or legally responsible.

4. _____ assures that high-quality diagnostic radiographs are produced.

5. Specific tests that are used to assure quality in dental x-ray equipment, supplies, and film processing are _____.

MULTIPLE CHOICE

Complete each question by circling the best answer.

1. What federal act requires persons who take radiographs to be trained and certified?
   a. OSHA
   b. CDC
   c. Consumer-Patient Radiation Health and Safety Act
   d. Bill of Rights

2. What type of agreement is necessary before exposing radiographs on a patient?

   a. Verbal consent
   b. Dentist's signature
   c. Written consent
   d. Medical approval

3. Under state laws, who is allowed to prescribe dental radiographs?

   a. Radiologist
   b. Specialist
   c. Physician
   d. Dentist

4. Who legally owns patient's dental radiographs?

   a. Patient
   b. Radiologist
   c. Dentist
   d. Physician

5. A way to assure that high-quality diagnostic radiographs are produced is by having:

   a. the best type of film.
   b. quality assurance.
   c. certified dental assistants.
   d. Kodak approval.

6. What are quality control tests?

   a. Specific tests that are used to monitor dental x-ray equipment, supplies, and film processing
   b. Specific tests that dental personnel must take and pass
   c. National boards for dentists
   d. Radiology certification

7. When should you check a box of film for freshness?

   a. Daily
   b. Monthly
   c. Monday morning
   d. Each time you open up a new box

8. Should you use a film cassette that has scratches?

   a. Yes
   b. No

9. What is one of the most critical areas in a quality control program?

   a. Patient consent
   b. Film mounting
   c. Film processing
   d. Use of PPE

10. What is the purpose of the coin test?

    a. To check the x-ray machine
    b. To check the safelight
    c. To check the processor
    d. To check the technique

11. How often should processing solutions be replenished?

    a. Daily
    b. Weekly
    c. Monthly
    d. Twice a year

12. Why are a reference radiograph and stepwedge used?

    a. To check the absorbed dose
    b. To check the processing technique
    c. To check the densities and contrast
    d. To check the radiolucency and radiopacity

13. How can you tell when the fixer is losing its strength?

    a. When films take longer to clear
    b. When films appear dark
    c. When films are black
    d. When films appear light

14. What is the purpose of a quality administration program?

    a. Deals with the credentialing of quality assurance program
    b. Deals with the management of the quality assurance program
    c. Deals with who takes the x-rays in the office
    d. Deals with being compensated more for taking x-rays

15. Which staff members need to be aware of the quality administration program?

    a. Dentist
    b. Dental assistant
    c. Dental hygienist
    d. All of the above

16. What surfaces must be covered with barriers?

    a. All surfaces during the procedure
    b. Any surfaces that are not easily cleaned and disinfected
    c. No surfaces should be covered with a barrier
    d. Only surfaces in the darkroom

17. What precautions should be taken when handling contaminated film?

    a. Wearing of overgloves
    b. Not walking around with film in your hand
    c. Use of a liquid sterilant
    d. Wiping saliva off film as soon as it is removed from the mouth

18. What personal protective equipment should the operator wear while exposing radiographs?

    a. Mask
    b. Eyewear
    c. Gloves
    d. Hair cover

CASE STUDY

A series of films has just been processed in the automatic processor, and something has happened to them. You take them to the viewbox, and all the films are dark. Dark films can be the result of various processing errors. Explain how the following causes can affect the processing of a film.

1. Time:
2. Solution strength:
3. Temperature:
4. Light leaks:
5. Improper fixation:
6. Paper left on film:

41 | Intraoral Radiography

SHORT ANSWER QUESTIONS

1. Describe the procedure for preparing a patient for dental radiographs.
2. Name and describe the two primary types of projections used in an intraoral technique.
3. Explain the advantages and disadvantages of the paralleling and bisection of the angle techniques.
4. Explain the basic principle of the paralleling technique.
5. Explain why a film holder is necessary with the paralleling technique.
6. State the five basic rules of the paralleling technique.
7. Label the parts of Rinn XCP instruments.
8. State the recommended vertical angulation for all bite-wing exposures.
9. State the basic rules for the bite-wing technique.
10. Describe the appearance of opened and overlapped contact areas on a dental radiograph.
11. State the basic rules of the bisecting technique.
12. Describe the film size used in the bisecting technique.
13. Describe correct vertical angulation.
14. Describe incorrect vertical angulation.
15. Describe the technique for exposing occlusal radiographs.
16. Describe techniques for managing the patient with a hypersensitive gag reflex.
17. Describe techniques for managing patients with physical and mental disabilities.

FILL IN THE BLANK

Select the best term from the list below and complete the following statements.

Alveolar bone
Bisection of the angle technique
Bite-wing film
Central ray
Contact areas
Crestal bone
Diagnostic quality
Interproximal

Intersecting
Long axis of the tooth
Open contacts
Parallel
Paralleling technique
Perpendicular
Right-angle

1. The _____ is an intraoral technique of exposing periapical films in which the teeth and film are parallel to each other.

2. The _____ is an intraoral technique of exposing periapical films in which the film and teeth create an angle that is bisected by the beam.

3. Radiographs with the proper images and optimum density, contrast, definition, and detail have good _____.

4. _____ is a term used to describe a space between two adjacent surfaces.

5. A _____ is the type of film used in the interproximal examination.

6. The bone that supports and encases the roots of the teeth is the _____.

7. The _____ is the coronal portion of alveolar bone found between the teeth.

8. An area of a tooth that touches an adjacent tooth in the same arch is the

   _____.

9. _____ appear on dental radiographs as thin radiolucent lines between adjacent teeth in the same arch.

10. An object is _____ if it is moving or lying in the same plane and always separated by the same distance.

11. _____ means to cut across or through.

12. Something is _____ if it intersects at or forms a right angle.

13. An angle of 90° formed by two lines perpendicular to each other is

    a _____.

14. The _____ is an imaginary line dividing the tooth longitudinally into two equal halves.

15. The _____ is the central portion of the primary beam of radiation.

MULTIPLE CHOICE

Complete each question by circling the best answer.

1. What technique is used for exposing radiographs?

   a. Digressive
   b. Parallel
   c. Bisection of angle
   d. b and c

2. Which technique do the American Academy of Oral and Maxillofacial Radiology and the American Association of Dental Schools recommend?

   a. Bisection of angle
   b. Parallel
   c. Intersection
   d. Dissection

3. Why is an exposure sequence important?

   a. So that areas of the mouth are not missed or retaken
   b. Guidelines have to be followed
   c. For proper mounting of film
   d. Keep up with them in the processing

4. When exposing films, in which area of the mouth should you begin?

   a. Maxillary right
   b. Mandibular anterior
   c. Mandibular left
   d. Maxillary anterior

5. Which exposure should be the first for posterior exposures?

   a. Maxillary molar
   b. Mandibular premolar
   c. Maxillary premolar
   d. Mandibular molar

6. Why is it not recommended to have the patient hold the film during exposure?

   a. Finger will get in the way of the image
   b. Dental assistant can not position the film properly
   c. Patient receives unnecessary radiation
   d. Does not meet with infection control standards

7. What type of film holder can be used in the bisecting angle technique?

   a. BAI
   b. EEZEE Grip
   c. Stabe
   d. All of the above

8. What error occurs when the horizontal angulation is incorrect?

   a. Elongation
   b. Overlapping
   c. Blurred
   d. Herringbone pattern

9. What error occurs when the vertical angulation is incorrect?

   a. Elongation
   b. Overlapping
   c. Foreshortening
   d. a and c

10. In the bisecting angle technique, how is the film placed in relation to the teeth?

    a. Parallel
    b. Far from the teeth
    c. Close to the teeth
    d. Opposite side of the arch

11. What is the purpose of bite-wing radiographs?

    a. View the occlusal third
    b. View the gingival third
    c. View the apex
    d. View the interproximal

12. What horizontal angulation should be used for bite-wing radiographs?

    a. –10 degrees
    b. +15 degrees
    c. +10 degrees
    d. –15 degrees

13. What size film is used in the occlusal technique?

    a. 1
    b. 2
    c. 3
    d. 4

14. When are occlusal radiographs indicated?

    a. Wide view of the arch
    b. To view the sinus
    c. For detection of interproximal decay
    d. For view of apex

15. For partially edentulous patients, how can you modify the technique for using a bite-block?

    a. Use of a larger size of film
    b. Use of a cotton roll
    c. Use of a partial
    d. Use of a custom tray

16. When exposing films on a pediatric patient, what analogy can you use to describe the tubehead?

    a. Space gun
    b. Alien machine
    c. Camera
    d. Tubehead

17. What changes must be made in the exposure factors when exposing radiographs on a pediatric patient?

    a. No changes are made
    b. Exposure factors must be reduced
    c. Exposure factors must be increased
    d. Depends if the patient is male or female

18. What size film is recommended for a pediatric patient with all primary dentition?

    a. 0
    b. 1
    c. 2
    d. 3

19. Where would you begin taking radiographs on a patient with a severe gag reflex?

    a. Maxillary anterior
    b. Mandibular molar
    c. Maxillary molar
    d. Mandibular anterior

20. What is a good diagnostic quality radiograph for endodontics?

    a. One that shows an impaction
    b. One that you can see interproximally
    c. One that you can see 5 mm beyond the apex
    d. One that shows the incisal edge

21. When mounting radiographs, where is the dot placed?

    a. Does not matter
    b. Facing away from you
    c. Facing down
    d. Facing up

22. Why is it important for the dental assistant to recognize normal anatomical landmarks?

    a. For diagnostic purposes
    b. For mounting of x-rays
    c. For quality control
    d. For identification of the patient

23. Why is it important to avoid retakes?

    a. Dentist will deduct from pay
    b. Unnecessary radiation exposure
    c. Deplete film quota
    d. Insurance will not pay for the procedure

MOUNTING EXERCISE

Located on the *Saunders Interactive Dental Office CD* is a series of mounting exercises for your practice. Begin the exercises using a 5-minute allowance. Time these exercises, and note how many errors are taken when placing these on the mount. Continue this exercise until you have your mounting skills down to 2 minutes with no errors.

42 | Extraoral and Digital Radiography

SHORT ANSWER QUESTIONS

1. Describe the purpose and uses of panoramic radiography.
2. Describe the equipment used in panoramic radiography.
3. Describe the steps for patient positioning in panoramic radiography.
4. Discuss the advantages and disadvantages of panoramic radiography.
5. Describe common errors made during patient preparation and positioning for panoramic radiography.
6. Describe the equipment used in extraoral radiography.
7. Identify the specific purpose of each of the extraoral film projections.
8. Describe the purposes and uses of extraoral radiography.
9. Describe the purpose and use of digital radiography.
10. Discuss the fundamentals of digital radiography.
11. List and describe the equipment used in digital radiography.
12. List and discuss the advantages and disadvantages of digital radiography.

FILL IN THE BLANKS

Select the best term from the list below and complete the following statements.

Charge-coupled device
Digital radiography
Digitize
Focal trough
Frankfort plane
Midsagittal plane
Sensor
Tomography

1. An imaginary three-dimensional curved zone that is horseshoe shaped and used to focus panoramic radiographs is the

   _____.

2. The _____ is the imaginary plane that passes through the top of the ear canal and the bottom of the eye socket.

3. The imaginary line that divides the patient's face into right and left sides is the

   _____.

4. _____ is a radiographic technique that allows imaging of one layer or section of the body while blurring images from structures in other planes.

5. A _____ is an image receptor found in the intraoral sensor.

6. To convert an image into a digital form that in turn can be processed by a computer is

   to _____.

7. A small detector that is placed intraorally to capture a radiographic image is the

   _____.

8. _____ is a filmless imaging system that uses a sensor to capture an image, break it into electronic pieces, and store it in a computer.

MULTIPLE CHOICE

Complete each question by circling the best answer.

1. When are extraoral radiographs needed?
   a. To detect decay
   b. To view large areas of the jaws or skull
   c. For a patient who gags
   d. When the processor is not working

2. What additional films might be needed to supplement a panoramic radiograph?

   a. Periapical
   b. Bite-wing
   c. Occlusal
   d. All of the above

3. A focal trough is:

   a. the area where the patient bites down.
   b. an imaginary horseshoe-shaped area used for jaw placement.
   c. where the patient looks during the process.
   d. earpieces used for positioning.

4. The purpose of extraoral radiographs is to:

   a. show a close-up image of something.
   b. prevent a patient from receiving too much radiation.
   c. provide an overall image of the skull and jaws.
   d. prevent a patient from having to place anything intraorally.

5. What type of device is added onto a panoramic unit?

   a. Cephalostat
   b. Hemostat
   c. Custom tray
   d. Dental dam

6. The purpose of a grid is to:

   a. increase the size of the image.
   b. reduce the amount of scatter radiation.
   c. hold the patient's head still.
   d. hold the film in place.

7. What type of imaging is best for soft tissues of the TMJ?

   a. Panorex
   b. Digital x-ray
   c. Cephalometric
   d. Computed tomograph

8. In digital radiography, what replaces the intraoral film?

   a. Bite-block
   b. Sensor
   c. Intensifying screen
   d. Cassette

9. How are sensors sterilized?

   a. Heat
   b. Moist
   c. Vapor
   d. Sensors cannot be sterilized

10. Which exposure technique is preferred when using digital radiography?

    a. Bite-wing
    b. Parallel
    c. Occlusal
    d. Bisection of the angle

CASE STUDY

Jeramy Davis is a 16-year-old male who is scheduled for an exam and consult today. Some of the problems that Jeramy exhibits are (1) class III occlusion, (2) crowding, and (3) recurrent decay with (4) slight gingivitis. In order for the dentist to proceed, a more detailed evaluation is required using radiographs.

1. What type of radiograph would reveal a class III occlusion?
2. What type of radiograph would reveal crowding?
3. What specialist should Jeramy be referred to for his class III occlusion and crowding?
4. What type of radiographs would reveal recurrent decay?
5. What type of radiograph would reveal gingivitis?

43 | Restorative and Esthetic Materials

SHORT ANSWER QUESTIONS

1. Discuss how a dental material is evaluated before being marketed to the profession.
2. List the properties of dental materials and how these affect their application.
3. Discuss the difference between direct and indirect restorative materials.
4. Describe the factors that affect how dental materials are manufactured for the oral cavity.
5. Describe the properties of amalgam and its application in restoring teeth.
6. Describe the properties of composite resin materials and their application in restoring teeth.
7. Describe the properties of glass ionomers and their application in restoring teeth.
8. Describe the properties of temporary restorative materials and their application in restoring teeth.
9. Discuss the use of tooth-whitening products.
10. Describe the properties of gold alloys and their application in restoring teeth.
11. Describe the properties of porcelain and its application in restoring teeth.

FILL IN THE BLANK

Select the best term from the list below and complete the following statements.

Adhere
Alloy
Amalgam
Auto-cure
Ceramic
Coupling agent
Cured
Esthetic
Filler
Force
Galvanic
Gold
Irregular
Malleability
Matrix

Microleakage
Palladium
Pestle
Platinum
Porcelain
Restorative
Retention
Spherical
Strain
Stress
Trituration
Viscosity
Wetting

1. _____ causes physical change through energy and strength.

2. A(n) _____ reaction is the effect of an electric shock when two metals touch.

3. _____ is a hard, brittle, heat-resistant, and corrosive-resistant material that resembles clay.

4. A(n) _____ is something that joins or connects two things together.

5. When a material is _____, it is preserved, or finished by a chemical or physical process.

6. To stick or glue two items together is to _____.

7. _____ is a soft, steel-white, tarnish-resistant metal that occurs naturally with platinum.

8. Something that restores or brings back to its natural appearance is called _____.

9. An object that moves vertically to pound or pulverize a material is a(n) _____.

10. _____ is a silver-white metal that does not corrode in air.

11. _____ is a hard, white, translucent ceramic made by firing pure clay and then glazing it.

12. _____ is an artistically pleasing and beautiful appearance.

13. A(n) _____ can be added to a material to fill pores, cracks, or holes.

14. _____ is a soft, yellow, corrosive-resistant metal used in making indirect restorations.

15. Particles that are _____ are not straight, uniform, or symmetrical.

16. A dental material that has _____ is capable of being shaped or formed without permanent damage.

17. The property of a liquid that causes it not to flow easily is its _____.

18. _____ is to cover or soak something with a liquid.

19. The chemical makeup of a material has a(n) _____ that allows the material to bind to a substance or to hold together.

20. A mixture of alloys with mercury becomes _____.

21. _____ refers to how a material hardens or sets by a chemical reaction of two materials.

22. A(n) _____ is a minute area where moisture and contaminates can enter.

23. A(n) _____ is a mixture of two or more metals.

24. _____ is the ability to retain or hold something in place.

25. Something that is round shaped is said to be _____.

26. _____ is to stretch or force something beyond its limits.

27. An applied force that strains or deforms something is added _____.

28. _____ is a method used to process dental materials.

MULTIPLE CHOICE

Complete each question by circling the best answer.

1. What professional organization evaluates a new dental material?
   a. FDA
   b. DDS
   c. ADA
   d. MDA

2. What type of reaction does a dental material undergo when there is distortion?
   a. Strain
   b. Stress
   c. Compression
   d. Distortion

3. What happens to a dental material when it is exposed to hot and then cold?
   a. Contraction and expansion
   b. Melting and hardening
   c. Galvanic reaction
   d. Strain and stress

4. Give an example of how galvanic action takes place.
   a. Salt within the saliva
   b. Leakage of a material
   c. Touching of two metals
   d. a and c

5. Select a property that is essential in the application of a dental material.

   a. Appearance
   b. Match the tooth color
   c. Retention
   d. Use of instruments

6. How does an auto-cured material harden or set?

   a. Air dry
   b. Chemical reaction
   c. Light
   d. Heat

7. Give the makeup of the alloy powder in amalgam.

   a. Porcelain, glass, zinc, and composite
   b. Gold, tin, silver, and aluminum
   c. Mercury, silver, zinc, and tin
   d. Silver, tin, copper, and zinc

8. Why is dental amalgam not placed in anterior teeth?

   a. Esthetics
   b. Not strong enough
   c. Hard to finish
   d. Retention

9. Most amalgams have a high copper content. What does copper provide to amalgam restorations?

   a. Strength
   b. Malleability
   c. Corrosion resistance
   d. a and c

10. Where do you dispose of amalgam scraps?

    a. Garbage
    b. Down the sink
    c. Under water or fixer solution
    d. In a biohazard bag

11. How is amalgam triturated?

    a. Mortar and pestle
    b. Amalgamator
    c. Paper pad and spatula
    d. Bowl and spatula

12. How long is sybraloy triturated?

    a. 3 seconds
    b. 7 seconds
    c. 13 seconds
    d. 20 seconds

13. Give the common term used to describe dimethacrylate.

    a. Alloy
    b. Composite resin
    c. Mercury
    d. BIS-GMA

14. What filler type of composite resin has the strongest makeup and is used most commonly for posterior restorations?

    a. Macrofilled
    b. Microfilled
    c. Monofilled
    d. Autofilled

15. When light-curing composite resins, what factor might require a longer curing time of the material?

    a. Tooth
    b. Depth of restoration
    c. Surface being restored
    d. Type of composite

16. What item is used to determine the color of composite for a procedure?

    a. Color palate
    b. Picture
    c. Shade guide
    d. Scanner

17. What would be the final step in finishing a composite resin?

    a. Diamond bur
    b. Sandpaper strip
    c. Polishing paste
    d. White stone

18. What does the abbreviation *IRM* stand for?

    a. Inside the restorative matrix
    b. Intermediate restorative material
    c. Interdental resin material
    d. International restorative material

19. What temporary restorative material may be selected for a class II cavity preparation?

    a. Composite
    b. Amalgam
    c. Permanent cement
    d. IRM

20. What material would you set up in the preparation for provisional coverage?

    a. IRM
    b. Acrylic
    c. Amalgam
    d. Alginate

21. How many drops of monomer of acrylic are recommended per tooth?

    a. 5
    b. 10
    c. 15
    d. 20

22. What are the three noble metals used in dentistry?

    a. Gold, palladium, and platinum
    b. Silver, tin, and zinc
    c. Mercury, copper, and tin
    d. Glass, porcelain, and fillers

23. What type of restoration is made in the dental laboratory?

    a. Direct restoration
    b. Provisional coverage
    c. Indirect restoration
    d. Temporary restoration

CASE STUDY

You are assisting in a restorative procedure for teeth #10 and #11. The patient record shows that the decay is at the gingival aspect on the facial surface of both teeth. The dentist has asked you to set up the dental dam for the procedure.

1. What cavity classification does this type of decay represent?
2. What type of restorative material would most likely be selected for teeth #10 and #11?
3. List the materials that would be set out for the application of the material specified when setting up for the procedure.
4. Why is it important to use a dental dam in this procedure?
5. How would this procedure be charted in a patient record?

44 | Dental Liners, Bases, and Bonding Systems

SHORT ANSWER QUESTIONS

1. Describe how the sensitivity of a tooth determines what kind of dental material is selected for a procedure.
2. Describe how and why cavity liners are used in the restoration process.
3. Describe how and why varnishes are used in the restoration process.
4. Describe how and why dentin sealers are used in the restoration process.
5. Describe how and why dental bases are used in the restoration process.
6. Describe the etching process of a tooth and its importance in the bonding procedure.
7. Describe the bonding systems and how they provide a better adaptation of a dental material to the tooth structure.

FILL IN THE BLANK

Select the best term from the list below and complete the following statements.

Desiccate
Etching
Eugenol
Hybrid
Insulating
Micromechanical
Obliterating
Polymerize
Protective
Retention
Sedative
Smear layer
Thermal

1. The _____ is a very thin layer of debris on newly prepared dentin.

2. _____ relates to heat.

3. A composite material that produces a similar outcome to its natural counterpart is called a(n) _____.

4. _____ is the means to prevent the passage of heat or electricity.

5. _____ is the process to cut into a surface by the use of an acid product.

6. _____ is the process of bonding two or more monomers.

7. _____ is a colorless liquid made from clove oil used for its soothing qualities.

8. _____ is the ability to provide protection.

9. _____ is an item that has all of the moisture removed, or dried.

10. _____ is the union of a material and structure with one another through minute cuttings.

11. _____ is the process of removing completely.

12. Some dental materials have a(n) _____ effect, which provides a soothing or calming effect.

13. _____ is the ability to hold or retain something.

MULTIPLE CHOICE

Complete each question by circling the best answer.

1. The purpose of a dental liner is to:
   a. make the restorative material look natural.
   b. protect the pulp from any type of irritation.
   c. create a mechanical lock of the dental material.
   d. cover the smear layer.

2. What tooth surface is calcium hydroxide placed on?

   a. Enamel
   b. Cementum
   c. Dentin
   d. Pulp

3. Which is *not* a unique characteristic of calcium hydroxide?

   a. Protects the tooth from chemical irritation
   b. Produces reparative dentin
   c. Compatible with all restorative materials
   d. Replaces the need for a dentin sealer

4. What is the main ingredient in varnish?

   a. Resin
   b. Acid
   c. Eugenol
   d. Sealant

5. Which material is contraindicated under composite resins and glass ionomer restorations?

   a. Etchant
   b. Calcium hydroxide
   c. Dentin sealer
   d. Varnish

6. Give another name associated with dentin sealer.

   a. Cement
   b. Desensitizer
   c. Etchant
   d. Base

7. What does the dentin sealer seal?

   a. Enamel rods
   b. Etched tags
   c. Dentin tubules
   d. Pulpal chambers

8. What does an insulating base provide?

   a. Protects the pulp from thermal shock
   b. Protects the pulp from moisture
   c. Helps soothe the pulp
   d. Protects the pulp from the restoration

9. What effects does eugenol have on the pulp?

   a. Irritant
   b. Soothing
   c. Protective
   d. Restorative

10. Where is a base applied in a cavity preparation?

    a. Proximal box
    b. Cavity walls
    c. Enamel margin
    d. Pulpal floor

11. What dental instrument is used to adapt a base into a cavity preparation?

    a. Explorer
    b. Hollenback
    c. Condenser
    d. Burnisher

12. What is the purpose of a dental bonding material?

    a. Sealer
    b. Bonds restorative materials to tooth structure
    c. Etchant
    d. Permanent restorative material

13. Give an example of enamel bonding.

    a. Composite resins
    b. Sealants
    c. Liner
    d. a and b

14. What must be removed from tooth structure for bonding material to reach dentin?

    a. Enamel
    b. Decay
    c. Smear layer
    d. Dentin tubules

15. Which sequence is recommended for the application of supplementary materials for a deep restoration?

    a. Liner, base, dentin sealer, bonding system
    b. Base, liner, dentin sealer, bonding system
    c. Bonding system, base, liner, dentin sealer
    d. Dentin sealer, base, bonding system, liner

CASE STUDY

Dr. Clark has completed the preparation of a class III on the distal surface of tooth #7. She has asked for you to prepare and ready the supplemental materials for placement. You inquire the depth of the preparation, and Dr. Clark indicates that it is moderately deep.

1. What type of final restorative material would most likely be selected for tooth #7?
2. What supplemental materials should be set up for this procedure?
3. How many steps will be required to complete the application of these supplemental materials?
4. What type of moisture control is used during the application of these materials?
5. In the application of these supplemental materials, are any of them legal for the expanded function assistant in your state? If so, what are they?

45 | Dental Cements

SHORT ANSWER QUESTIONS

1. Describe luting cements and the difference between permanent and temporary.
2. Discuss the factors that influence luting cements.
3. List the five cements discussed in the chapter, and describe their similarities and differences.

FILL IN THE BLANK

Select the best term from the list below and complete the following statements.

   Cement
   Exothermic
   Luting agent
   Provisional
   Retard
   Spatulate

1. To _____ is to mix using a spatula type instrument.

2. _____ refers to the release of heat from a chemical reaction.

3. A(n) _____ is a temporary type of crown or bridge used for a short time.

4. A dental material that is used to temporarily or permanently hold an indirect restoration in place is a(n)

   _____.

5. To _____ is to slow down the process of something.

6. A cementlike substance used to seal a surface is a(n) _____.

MULTIPLE CHOICE

Complete each question by circling the best answer.

1. Another name for a permanent cement is a:

   a. liner.
   b. luting agent.
   c. resin.
   d. base.

2. When would temporary cement be used?

   a. Composite restoration
   b. Sealants
   c. Amalgam restoration
   d. Provisional coverage

3. What variable affects the addition or loss of water in a material?

   a. Time
   b. Speed of spatulation
   c. Humidity
   d. Moisture control

4. What type of ZOE is used for permanent cementation?

   a. Type I
   b. Type II
   c. Type III
   d. Type IV

5. What type of mixing pad is ZOE mixed on?

   a. Treated paper pad
   b. Glass
   c. Plastic
   d. Cardboard

6. How is Temp bond supplied?

   a. Powder and liquid
   b. Paste and powder
   c. Two tubes of paste
   d. Two liquids

7. The main component in the liquid of zinc phosphate is:

   a. hydrogen peroxide.
   b. zinc oxide.
   c. resin.
   d. phosphoric acid.

8. How do you dissipate the heat from zinc phosphate during the mixing process?

   a. Cool the spatula
   b. Use a cool glass slab
   c. Turn the temperature down in the room
   d. Chill the material

9. What size of powder increment is first brought into the liquid of zinc phosphate when mixing?

   a. Smallest
   b. Medium
   c. Half of the material
   d. Largest

10. How do you load a crown with permanent cement?

    a. Overfill
    b. Fill
    c. Line
    d. Occlusal surface only

11. How is polycarboxylate cement liquid supplied?

    a. Tube
    b. Squeeze bottle
    c. Calibrated syringe
    d. b and c

12. How should polycarboxylate cement appear after the mixing process?

    a. Dull
    b. Glossy
    c. Streaky
    d. Clear

13. Can glass ionomer cements be used as a restoration?

    a. Yes
    b. No

14. What ingredient in the powder of glass ionomer cement helps in inhibiting recurrent decay?

    a. Zinc
    b. Composite resin
    c. Iron
    d. Calcium

15. Can resin cements be used under metal castings?

    a. Yes
    b. No

16. What procedure should be completed before cementation with composite resin cement?

    a. Coronal polishing
    b. Placement of a sealant
    c. Etching and bonding
    d. Placement of a liner

CASE STUDY

Dr. Stewart will be cementing four stainless steel crowns today on a 10-year-old patient. She has indicated that Duralon will be the cement of choice.

1. Are stainless steel crowns permanent or temporary?
2. What type of cement is Duralon?
3. List what is needed for the setup.
4. Describe the mixing technique for this cement.
5. How would the cement be cleaned up from around the cemented crown?

46 | Impression Materials

SHORT ANSWER QUESTIONS

1. List the three types of impressions taken in a dental office.
2. Describe the types of impression trays and their characteristics of use.
3. Discuss hydrocolloid impression materials and describe their use, mixing techniques, and application of material.
4. Discuss elastomeric impression materials and describe their use, mixing techniques, and application of material.
5. Describe the importance of an occlusal registration and its use in a procedure.

FILL IN THE BLANK

Select the best term from the list below and complete the following statements.

Agar
Alginate
Base
Border molding
Catalyst
Centric
Colloid
Elastomeric
Extrude
Hydro
Imbibition
Occlusal
Registration
Syneresis
Tempering
Viscosity

1. _____ is a gelatin-like material.

2. _____ is the process of using your fingers to achieve a closer adaptation of the edges of an impression.

3. A(n) _____ material has elastic properties from rubber.

4. A fundamental ingredient of a material is the _____.

5. To have something _____ is having an object centered, such as your maxillary teeth centered over your mandibular teeth.

6. _____ is a gelatin-type material derived from seaweed.

7. _____ is the loss of water, causing shrinkage.

8. _____ is to bring a material to a desired consistency.

9. _____ describes a material with a high resistance to flow.

10. _____ is the material of choice used in dentistry for preliminary impressions.

11. To push or force out is to _____.

12. _____ means water.

13. A(n) _____ is a reproduction of someone's bite using wax or elastomeric material.

14. A(n) _____ is a substance that modifies or increases a rate of a chemical reaction.

15. _____ is the absorption of water, causing an object to swell.

MULTIPLE CHOICE

Complete each question by circling the best answer.

1. An impression is a:

   a. negative reproduction.
   b. mirror image.
   c. positive reproduction.
   d. duplication.

2. Of the 3 classification of impressions, which could the expanded function assistant legally take?

   a. Preliminary
   b. Final
   c. Bite registration
   d. a or c

3. Which of the 3 classification of impressions is used for occlusal relationship?

   a. Preliminary
   b. Final
   c. Bite registration
   d. Temporary

4. What type of tray covers half of the arch?

   a. Anterior
   b. Quadrant
   c. Full
   d. Custom

5. What type of tray allows impression material to mechanically lock on?

   a. Metal
   b. Plastic
   c. Custom
   d. Perforated

6. What kind of tray is most commonly used for taking final impressions?

   a. Metal
   b. Plastic
   c. Custom
   d. Perforated

7. What is used to extend the length of a tray?

   a. Rope wax
   b. Impression material
   c. Border molding
   d. Boxing wax

8. The organic substance of hydrocolloid materials is:

   a. tree bark.
   b. volcanic ash.
   c. seaweed.
   d. mud.

9. Why might a fast-set alginate be selected for taking a preliminary impression?

   a. Patient is late for the appointment
   b. Patient has a strong gag reflex
   c. Patient does not like the taste
   d. To keep patient from talking

10. What is the water-powder ratio for taking a maxillary impression?

    a. One scoop of powder to the first level of water
    b. Two scoops of powder to the second level of water
    c. Three scoops of powder to the third level of water
    d. Four scoops of powder to the fourth level of water

11. *Hydro* means:

    a. air.
    b. mass.
    c. water.
    d. temperature.

12. Another name for irreversible hydrocolloid is:

    a. alginate.
    b. elastomeric.
    c. polyether.
    d. polysulfide.

13. How is irreversible hydrocolloid mixed?

    a. Glass slab
    b. Mixing bowl
    c. Paper pad
    d. Automix system

14. Where should reversible hydrocolloid be kept before taking an impression?

    a. Refrigerator
    b. Oven
    c. Room temperature
    d. Conditioning bath

15. Elastomeric materials are used for what type of impression?

    a. Final
    b. Preliminary
    c. Bite registration
    d. Temporary

16. How are elastomeric materials supplied?

    a. Paste
    b. Cartridge
    c. Putty
    d. All of the above

17. Which viscosity of final impression material is first applied to the teeth?

    a. Light
    b. Medium
    c. Heavy

18. Another term for polysulfide is:

    a. polyether.
    b. rubber base.
    c. silicone.
    d. alginate.

19. How is light-body final impression material placed on a prepared tooth?

    a. Spatula
    b. Perforated tray
    c. Syringe
    d. Custom tray

20. What system completes the mixing of final impression material for you?

    a. Vibrator
    b. Spatula and pad
    c. Triturator
    d. Auto-mix

21. What is most commonly used for taking a bite registration?

    a. Base plate wax
    b. Alginate
    c. Silicone
    d. Rubber base

22. What type of tray would most commonly be selected when using ZOE bite registration paste?

    a. Perforated tray
    b. Metal tray
    c. Gauze bite tray
    d. Water-cooled tray

23. How is wax prepared before placement in the patient's mouth for a bite registration?

    a. Molded
    b. Cooled
    c. Placed in a tray
    d. Warmed

CASE STUDY

Dr. Clark has asked you to take a maxillary and mandibular preliminary impression on the next patient for the fabrication of bleaching trays.

1. What impression material will be selected to take preliminary impressions?
2. Describe the setup that is required for taking these impressions.
3. Describe the mixing technique for taking this type of impression.
4. Is there any specific area of the mouth that is critical when taking this type of impression?
5. What will you do with these impressions once they are taken?

47 | Laboratory Materials and Procedures

SHORT ANSWER QUESTIONS

1. Discuss the safety precautions that should be taken in the dental lab.
2. List the types of equipment found in a dental lab and their use.
3. Describe dental models and how they are used in dentistry.
4. Discuss gypsum products and their use in making dental models.
5. Describe the three types of custom impression trays and their use in dentistry.
6. Describe the types of dental waxes and their use in dentistry.

FILL IN THE BLANK

Select the best term from the list below and complete the following statements.

Anatomic
Articulator
Crystallization
Dihydrate
Dimensionally
Facebow
Gypsum
Hemihydrate
Homogeneous
Lathe
Model
Monomer
Polymer
Slurry
Stable
Volatile

1. A material that is _____ is resistant to change.

2. A material is to be mixed

_____, with a uniform quality and consistency throughout.

3. A(n) _____ is a machine used for cutting or polishing of dental appliances.

4. _____ is a mineral that is used in the formation of plaster of Paris and stone.

5. A substance is said to be _____ when it can evaporate easily and is very explosive.

6. Relating to gypsum products, a(n)

_____ indicates that there are two parts of water to every part of calcium sulfate.

7. If you measure an object's width, height, and length, it is said to be

_____ sound.

8. The _____ is the portion of an articulator that is used to measure the upper teeth and compare to the temporomandibular joint.

9. A(n) _____ is the compounds of many molecules.

10. _____ is a chemical process in which crystals form a structure.

11. _____ is the removal of one-half part of water to one part of calcium sulfate forming the powder product of gypsum.

12. A(n) _____ is a replica of the maxillary and mandibular arches made from an impression.

13. _____ is the anatomy portion of an object.

14. A dental laboratory device that simulates the movement of the mandible and the temporomandibular joint when models of the dental arches are attached is the

    _____.

15. A(n) _____ is a molecule that when combined with others forms a polymer.

16. _____ is a mixture of gypsum and water used in the finishing of models.

MULTIPLE CHOICE

Complete each question by circling the best answer.

1. Where would the dental lab be located in a dental office?

    a. Treatment area
    b. Reception area
    c. Separate space away from patients
    d. Dentist's office

2. Which specialty practices might have a more extensive lab?

    a. Oral surgery
    b. Fixed prosthodontics
    c. Orthodontics
    d. b and c

3. Which would be an example of a contaminated item in the dental lab?

    a. Model trimmer
    b. Lathe
    c. Impression
    d. Sink

4. What piece of equipment is used to grind away plaster or stone?

    a. Model trimmer
    b. Lathe
    c. Bunsen burner
    d. Bab handpiece

5. What piece of equipment does the dentist use to determine centric relation on a diagnostic model?

    a. Vibrator
    b. Model trimmer
    c. Articulator
    d. Bunsen burner

6. The size of wax spatula most commonly used in the lab is a:

    a. number 1.
    b. number 3.
    c. number 5.
    d. number 7.

7. Another name for a dental model is a:

    a. die.
    b. impression.
    c. cast.
    d. waxup.

8. What dental material is used to fabricate dental models?

    a. Hydrocolloid
    b. Gypsum
    c. Elastomeric
    d. Wax

9. Which form of gypsum would be used to fabricate a die for making an indirect restoration?

    a. Plaster
    b. Stone
    c. High-strength stone

10. What is the water/powder ratio of plaster for pouring a model?

    a. 50/100
    b. 75/50
    c. 100/50
    d. 150/30

11. When mixing gypsum materials, how are the powder and water incorporated?

    a. Add water and powder at the same time
    b. Add water to the powder
    c. Add powder to the water
    d. Does not matter

12. How are gypsum materials mixed?

    a. Spatula and rubber bowl
    b. Spatula and paper pad
    c. Auto-mix
    d. Amalgamator

13. What are the parts of a dental model?

    a. Anatomic
    b. Art
    c. Skeletal
    d. a and b

14. When pouring an impression, where do you begin placing the gypsum material in a maxillary impression?

    a. Anterior teeth
    b. Palatal
    c. Most posterior tooth
    d. Premolar teeth

15. How long should you wait before you separate the model from the impression?

    a. 15 to 20 minutes
    b. 30 to 45 minutes
    c. 40 to 60 minutes
    d. 24 hours

16. Which of the two models (maxillary or mandibular) will you begin trimming first?

    a. Maxillary
    b. Smallest model
    c. Mandibular
    d. Largest model

17. What is one specific area on models where they are trimmed differently?

    a. Heels
    b. Buccal surfaces
    c. Base
    d. Anterior portion

18. What should be placed between the two models when trimming them together?

    a. Piece of material
    b. Wax bite
    c. Hydrocolloid material
    d. Gauze squares

19. Of the three types of custom trays discussed, which technique uses a volatile hazardous material?

    a. Acrylic resin
    b. Light-cured resin
    c. Thermoplastic resin
    d. Composite resin

20. What type of custom tray is made for a vital bleaching procedure?

    a. Acrylic resin
    b. Light-cured resin
    c. Thermoplastic resin
    d. Composite resin

21. Acrylic resin is supplied as:

    a. powder and liquid.
    b. tubes of paste.
    c. auto-mix.
    d. putty

22. What type of wax is used to form a wall around a preliminary impression when pouring it up?

    a. Rope wax
    b. Boxing wax
    c. Inlay wax
    d. Baseplate wax

23. To extend an impression tray, what type of wax would you use?

    a. Rope wax
    b. Boxing wax
    c. Inlay wax
    d. Baseplate wax

24. What type of wax would you use to get a patient's bite?

    a. Rope wax
    b. Boxing wax
    c. Inlay wax
    d. Baseplate wax

CASE STUDY

It is 4:30 in the afternoon, and Dr. Campbell has asked you to take preliminary impressions on a patient. The study models from these impressions will be used for a case presentation.

1. How are preliminary impressions cared for prior to taking them to the dental lab?
2. Due to the time of day, you ask Dr. Campbell if you can wait till tomorrow morning and pour them up. What would be her response, and why?
3. Because these models will be used for a case presentation, which gypsum material would provide a more professional presentation?
4. How will you remove any beads of gypsum and fill any voids for a more professional appearance?
5. How will you polish the finished model?

48 | Restorative Dentistry

SHORT ANSWER QUESTIONS

1. Describe the process and principles of cavity preparation.
2. Discuss the differences that occur when assisting with an amalgam and composite restoration.
3. Explain why retention pins would be selected for a complex procedure.
4. Describe the circumstances that call for placement of an intermediate restoration.
5. Describe the procedure of composite veneers.
6. Describe tooth-whitening techniques and the role of the dental assistant in these procedures.

FILL IN THE BLANK

Select the best term from the list below and complete the following statements.

Axial wall
Cavity
Cavity wall
Convenience form
Diastema
Operative
Outline form
Preparation
Pulpal wall
Resistance
Restoration
Retention
Veneer

1. A dental material that is used to restore a tooth to function is termed a(n)

   _____.

2. An internal surface of a cavity preparation is the _____.

3. The dentist will place a(n)

   _____ in the cavity preparation to hold a restorative material within the preparation.

4. A space between two teeth is termed a(n)

   _____.

5. A(n) _____ is a thin layer of restorative material used to correct a tooth surface.

6. A(n) _____ is a pitted area in a tooth caused by decay.

7. _____ allows the dentist an easier way in restoring a tooth.

8. A(n) _____ is a surface of a cavity preparation that is perpendicular to the pulp of a tooth.

9. The _____ is the design of how the tooth is prepared by the dentist to be restored.

10. _____ is a means of maintaining a restorative material within the preparation.

11. A(n) _____ procedure is the type of procedure that restores a tooth.

12. The _____ is a specific shape of a cavity preparation that the dentist uses in the restoration of a tooth.

13. A(n) _____ is an internal surface of a cavity preparation that is positioned in the same vertical direction as the pulp is in the tooth.

MULTIPLE CHOICE

Complete each question by circling the best answer.

1. What is restorative dentistry often called?
   a. Fillings
   b. Operative dentistry
   c. Prosthetic dentistry
   d. Surgical dentistry

2. A decayed tooth is also referred to as a(n):

   a. abscess.
   b. hole.
   c. preparation.
   d. cavity.

3. The process of removing decay is known as:

   a. cavity preparation.
   b. drill and fill.
   c. extraction.
   d. restoration.

4. What wall of the cavity preparation is perpendicular to the long axis of the tooth?

   a. Proximal wall
   b. Pulpal wall
   c. External wall
   d. Marginal wall

5. Where would you find a class I restoration in the mouth?

   a. Occlusal surface
   b. Buccal surface of a posterior tooth
   c. Lingual surface of an anterior tooth
   d. All of the above

6. How many surfaces can a class II restoration affect?

   a. One
   b. Two
   c. Three
   d. b and c

7. Which tooth could have a class II restoration placed?

   a. Tooth #8
   b. Tooth #13
   c. Tooth #22
   d. Tooth #27

8. What restorative material would you set up for a class IV restorative procedure?

   a. Composite resin
   b. Amalgam
   c. Veneer
   d. Bleaching

9. What kind of moisture control is recommended for class III and IV procedures?

   a. Cotton rolls
   b. 2 × 2 gauze
   c. Dental dam
   d. Saliva ejector

10. What population has a higher incidence of class V lesions?

    a. Children
    b. Teenagers
    c. Adults
    d. Older adults

11. Why would an intermediate restoration be placed?

    a. Health of tooth
    b. Waiting for permanent restoration
    c. Financial reasons
    d. All of the above

12. What tooth surface would most commonly receive a veneer?

    a. Lingual
    b. Facial
    c. Distal
    d. Incisal

13. The types of veneers that are placed are:

    a. direct-composite resin.
    b. indirect-porcelain.
    c. amalgam.
    d. a and b

14. Indications for having the tooth-whitening procedure are:

    a. extrinsic stains.
    b. aged teeth.
    c. intrinsic stains.
    d. all of the above

15. What is used to hold the tooth-whitening gel on the teeth?

    a. Thermoplastic tray
    b. Toothbrush
    c. Gauze tray
    d. Molded wax

16. The main ingredient of tooth-whitening products is:

    a. carbamide peroxide.
    b. phosphoric acid.
    c. hydrogen peroxide.
    d. a and c

17. What side effect may the patient experience during tooth whitening?

    a. Redness
    b. Fever
    c. Hypersensitivity
    d. Decay

CASE STUDY

Your next patient is scheduled to have a mesial/occlusal restoration placed in tooth #19.

1. What type of restorative material would most commonly be placed in this type of restoration for this specific tooth?
2. You will be preparing the dental dam for this procedure. Dr. Campbell prefers to have one tooth distal to the opposite canine isolated. What teeth will be involved in the isolation for this procedure?
3. What type of matrix system will be set up for this procedure?
4. What supplemental materials will you set out for this procedure?
5. After completion of the procedure, how would it be charted in the patient record?

49 | Matrix Systems for Restorative Dentistry

SHORT ANSWER QUESTIONS

1. Describe the need for a matrix system in the restoration of a class II, III, and IV procedure.
2. Describe the type of matrices used for posterior restorations.
3. Describe the type of matrices used for composite restorations.
4. Discuss the purpose and use of a wedge.
5. Discuss alternative methods of matrix systems used in the restorative dentistry.

FILL IN THE BLANK

Select the best term from the list below and complete the following statements.

Automatrix
Celluloid strip
Cupping
Matrix
Mylar
Overhang
Palodent
Universal retainer
Wedge

1. _____ is another name for a clear plastic strip that provides a temporary wall for the restoration of an anterior tooth.

2. Excess restorative material extending beyond the cavity margin is a(n)

   _____.

3. A plastic strip that provides a temporary wall for the restoration of an anterior tooth

   is the _____.

4. _____ is a term used when a tooth surface is concave and has not been contoured properly.

5. A(n) _____ is a wooden or plastic triangular-shaped item placed in the embrasure to provide the contour needed when restoring a class II restoration.

6. A(n) _____ is a band that provides a temporary wall to a tooth structure in order to restore the proximal contours and contact to its normal shape and function.

7. A(n) _____ is a small oval-shaped matrix made of stainless steel used interproximally during tooth restoration.

8. The _____ is a matrix system designed to establish a temporary wall for tooth restoration without using a retainer.

9. The _____ is used in dentistry to hold a matrix band in place during the restoration of a class II.

MULTIPLE CHOICE

Complete each question by circling the best answer.

1. Which classification would use a matrix system?
   a. I
   b. III
   c. V
   d. VI

2. The plural word for matrix is:

   a. matrixes.
   b. martinis.
   c. matrices.
   d. martins.

3. What is used to hold a posterior matrix band in position?

   a. Cotton pliers
   b. 110 pliers
   c. Wedge
   d. Universal retainer

4. When placing a matrix band into position, where is the smaller circumference of the band positioned?

   a. Gingival
   b. Occlusal
   c. Facial
   d. Lingual

5. What instrument can be used to thin and contour a matrix band?

   a. Condenser
   b. Explorer
   c. 110 pliers
   d. Burnisher

6. What additional item is used in the matrix system to reestablish a proper interproximal contact of the newly placed material?

   a. Retraction cord
   b. Wedge
   c. Explorer
   d. Articulating paper

7. What can improper wedge placement result in?

   a. Overfilling
   b. Cupping
   c. Overhang
   d. b and c

8. What matrix system could be an alternative to the Universal retainer?

   a. Celluloid strip
   b. Dental dam
   c. Stainless steel crown
   d. Automatrix

9. Why are metal matrix bands contraindicated with the use of composite resin materials?

   a. Do not fit around anterior teeth properly
   b. Cannot contour a metal band properly
   c. Metal can scratch some composite resins
   d. Keeps the dentist from seeing the preparation

10. Another term for the clear matrix is:

    a. celluloid.
    b. sandpaper strip.
    c. mylar strip.
    d. a and c

CASE STUDY

You are assisting in the restoration of tooth #29. The tooth is charted to have an MOD amalgam. During the preparation of the tooth, the dentist removes an extensive amount of tooth structure on the mesial facial cusp. The cavity preparation is now below the gingival margin, creating a large preparation.

1. What type of matrix system should be set up?
2. Because the preparation has changed, are there any changes that need to be made in the setup? If so, what are they?
3. How will the matrix band be adapted for the preparation mentioned above?
4. How many wedges will be used, and from what direction will they be inserted?
5. Could any other matrix system be used for this procedure? If so, what is it?

50 | Fixed Prosthodontics

SHORT ANSWER QUESTIONS

1. List the indications and contraindications for a fixed prosthesis.
2. Identify the steps for a diagnostic work-up.
3. Describe the role of the laboratory technician.
4. Describe the differences between full crowns, inlays, onlays, and veneer crowns.
5. Identify the components of a fixed bridge.
6. Describe the uses of porcelain for fixed prosthodontics.
7. Describe the preparation and placement of a cast crown.
8. Discuss the uses of core buildups, pins, and posts in crown retention.
9. Describe the use of retraction cord before taking a final impression.
10. Describe the function of provisional coverage for a crown or fixed bridge.
11. Give home care instructions for a permanent fixed prosthesis.

FILL IN THE BLANK

Select the best term from the list below and complete the following statements.

Abutment
Articulator
Bevel
Cast post
Chamfer
Core
Die
Fixed bridge
Full crown
Gingival retraction
Hypertrophied
Infuser
Inlay
Investment material
Master cast
Onlay
Opaquer
PFM
Pontic
Prosthetic
Resin-bonded bridge
Shade guide
Shoulder
Solder joint
Three-quarter crown
Unit
Veneer

1. The enamel margin of a crown preparation is the _____.

2. A(n) _____ is a metal support fitted into the root canal of an endodontically treated tooth to improve the retention of a cast restoration.

3. The _____ is the portion of a post and core that extends above the tooth structure.

4. The _____ is a replica of the prepared portion of a tooth used in the laboratory during the making of a cast restoration.

5. A(n) _____ can be a tooth, a root, or an implant used for the retention of a fixed or removable prosthesis.

6. A dental laboratory device that simulates the movements of the mandible and temporomandibular joint is the

   _____.

7. A fixed prosthetic with artificial teeth that are supported by attaching them to natural teeth is called a(n) _____.

8. _____ displaces gingival tissues away from the tooth.

9. The term _____ describes a tapered finish line of the margin at the cervical area of a tooth preparation.

10. A(n) _____ is a cast restoration that covers the entire anatomic crown of the tooth.

11. A cast restoration designed to restore a class II restoration is a(n)

    _____.

12. _____ means overgrown tissue.

13. A syringe that pushes hemostatic solution onto the gingival retraction cord is a(n)

    _____.

14. A(n) _____ is a cast that is created from a final impression used to construct baseplates, bite rims, wax setups, and finished prosthesis.

15. _____ is a special gypsum product that is able to withstand extreme heat.

16. The _____ is an artificial tooth that replaces a natural missing tooth.

17. The _____ is a type of indirect restoration in which a thin porcelain material is fused to the facial portion of a gold crown.

18. A(n) _____ is a layer of tooth-colored material either bonded or cemented to the prepared facial surface of a tooth.

19. The _____ is a cast restoration designed to restore the occlusal crown and proximal surfaces of a posterior tooth.

20. A(n) _____, also known as a Maryland bridge, has winglike projections that are bonded to the lingual surface of the adjacent teeth.

21. A(n) _____ is a resin material placed under a porcelain restoration to prevent the discoloration of the tooth from showing through.

22. A(n) _____ is a replacement for a missing body part.

23. A(n) _____ is a cast restoration that covers the anatomical crown of a tooth except for the facial or buccal portion.

24. The _____ are the margins of a tooth preparation for a cast restoration.

25. A(n) _____ is where two metal objects are united, such as on a bridge.

26. Each single component of the fixed bridge is considered a(n) _____.

27. The _____ is an accessory item that contains different shades of teeth, used to match a person's color of teeth for the laboratory technician.

MULTIPLE CHOICE

Complete each question by circling the best answer.

1. Fixed prosthodontics is commonly referred to as:

    a. operative.
    b. crown and bridge.
    c. dentures.
    d. prosthetics.

2. What would be a contraindication for a patient receiving fixed prosthodontics?

    a. Overweight
    b. Over the age of 60
    c. Poor oral hygiene
    d. Poor personal hygiene

3. What does the dentist use to reduce the height and contour of a tooth for a casting?

    a. Hand-cutting instrument
    b. Sandpaper disk
    c. Model trimmer
    d. Rotary instruments

4. If a tooth is nonvital, what is fabricated and placed into the pulp for better retention of a crown?

   a. Post and core
   b. Root canal filling
   c. Abutment
   d. Pontic

5. What is used during a crown and bridge preparation to displace gingival tissue?

   a. Cotton rolls
   b. Dental dam
   c. Gingival retraction cord
   d. Explorer

6. What astringent is applied to the retraction cord that can control bleeding?

   a. Hydrogen peroxide
   b. Epinephrine
   c. Disinfectant
   d. Coumadin

7. Another term used for overgrown tissue is:

   a. hyperthyroid.
   b. hyperplasia.
   c. hypertrophied.
   d. b and c

8. What type of impression is taken for the preparation of a crown?

   a. Preliminary
   b. Final
   c. Secondary
   d. Wax bites

9. How does the dentist tell the laboratory technician what kind of crown is needed?

   a. Conference call
   b. Fax the information
   c. Lab prescription
   d. Copy of the patient record

10. The laboratory technician prepares an exact replica of the prepared tooth. What is this replica called?

    a. Model
    b. Die
    c. Temporary
    d. Impression

11. What material does the lab tech use to create a pattern for the casting?

    a. Hydrocolloid
    b. Acrylic resin
    c. Composite
    d. Wax

12. What does the patient wear on the prepared tooth while the lab is making the crown or bridge?

    a. Stainless steel crown
    b. Provisional
    c. Wax
    d. Intermediate restorative material

13. Who in the dental office can legally permanently cement a crown or bridge?

    a. Dentist
    b. Hygienist
    c. Assistant
    d. Laboratory technician

14. How many appointments does it usually take for the dentist to deliver a fixed bridge?

    a. One
    b. Two
    c. Three
    d. b or c

15. What accessory is used to help in flossing a bridge?

    a. Waterpik
    b. Rubber tip
    c. Floss threader
    d. Electric toothbrush

16. How does the laboratory technician secure each unit of a bridge together?

    a. Permanent cement
    b. Bonding
    c. Light cure
    d. Solder

CASE STUDY

Mandy Moore needs a three-unit bridge on teeth #11 through #13. But due to prolonged neglect of her dental needs, Mandy must first go through a series of dental appointments to correct oral hygiene and restorative problems.

1. What hygiene problems might interfere with Mandy's having a bridge placed?
2. What type of bridge might be recommended for the teeth affected?
3. Which teeth are the pontic(s) and which are the abutment(s) for the discussed bridge?
4. Describe the type of provisional that would best suit this case.
5. Chart the following procedure with the type of bridge that was described in question number 2.

51 | Provisional Coverage

SHORT ANSWER QUESTIONS

1. Discuss the indications for provisional coverage for a crown or fixed bridge preparation.
2. Describe the types of provisional coverage.
3. Discuss the role of the expanded function dental assistant in the making of a provisional.
4. Identify home care instructions for provisional coverage.

FILL IN THE BLANK

Select the best term from the list below and complete the following statements.

Aluminum crown
Custom provisional
Polycarbonate crown
Preformed
Provisional

1. A(n) _____ is a provisional that is designed from a preliminary impression or thermoplastic tray resembling the tooth being prepared.

2. A(n) _____ is temporary coverage made for crown or bridge preparations to be worn during cast preparation.

3. An object that is already shaped in the appearance needed is

   _____.

4. The _____ is a thin aluminum shell used for provisional coverage of posterior teeth.

5. A(n) _____ is a provisional that is tooth colored and used for anterior teeth.

MULTIPLE CHOICE

Complete each question by circling the best answer.

1. A temporary covering for a crown or bridge is referred to as a(n):

   a. interim.
   b. provisional.
   c. crown.
   d. tray.

2. How long does a patient normally wear a provisional?

   a. 2 to 4 weeks
   b. 2 to 4 months
   c. 6 months
   d. 1 year

3. Who in the dental office can legally fabricate and cement a provisional?

   a. Dentist
   b. Assistant
   c. Hygienist
   d. All of the above

4. What type of provisional can be the most natural looking?

   a. Polycarbonate
   b. Aluminum
   c. Preformed acrylic
   d. Custom

5. What type of provisional would be selected for anterior teeth?

   a. Polycarbonate
   b. Aluminum
   c. Preformed acrylic
   d. a and c

6. What is required before preparation of the tooth in making a custom provisional?

   a. Preliminary impression
   b. Placement of gingival retraction cord
   c. Post and core
   d. Anesthesia

7. What type of dental material is used in making a custom provisional?

   a. Hydrocolloid
   b. Silicone
   c. Acrylic resin
   d. Amalgam

8. What is used to trim or contour an aluminum crown?

    a. Sandpaper disk
    b. Crown and bridge scissors
    c. Lathe
    d. Model trimmer

9. Does a polycarbonate crown remain on a prepared tooth, or is it just a mold for the provisional?

    a. Remains on the prepared tooth
    b. Mold for the material
    c. Either
    d. Not used as a provisional

10. Where is the mixed acrylic resin placed before seating it on the prepared tooth?

    a. On the prepared tooth
    b. In the impression
    c. In the thermo plastic tray
    d. b or c

CASE STUDY

You have been asked to make a provisional for tooth #30.

1. What type of provisional would most commonly be made for this tooth?
2. Describe two ways in which you can make a custom provisional.
3. After removing the provisional from the prepared tooth, you notice that the margins are not within 1 mm of the margin. What is your plan of action in improving the provisional so that it fits properly?
4. Once you have the provisional fitting properly, what is the next step before cementing the provisional?
5. What will you set up for cementation of the provisional? Describe the steps in the cement removal of the provisional.

52 | Removable Prosthodontics

SHORT ANSWER QUESTIONS

1. Differentiate between a partial and full denture.
2. Name indications and contraindications for removable partial and full dentures.
3. List the components of a partial denture.
4. List the components of a full denture.
5. Describe the steps in the construction of a removable partial denture.
6. Identify home care instructions for removable partial and full dentures.
7. Identify the process of relining or repairing a partial or full denture.

FILL IN THE BLANK

Select the best term from the list below and complete the following statements.

Alveoplasty
Articulator
Baseplate
Border molding
Centric relation
Connectors
Coping
Edentulous
Festooning
Flange
Framework
Frenum attachment
Full denture
Genial tubercles
Immediate denture
Lateral excursion
Mastication
Mylohyoid ridge
Oblique ridge
Occlusal rim
Partial denture
Post dam
Pressure points
Protrusion
Rebasing
Relining
Resorbed
Rest
Retainer
Retromolar pad
Retrusion
Surgical
Template
Tori
Tuberosities

1. A(n) _____ is a clear plastic tray that represents the alveolus as it should appear after teeth have been extracted.

2. _____ is abnormal growth of bone in a specific area.

3. _____ are rounded areas on the outer surface of the maxillary bones in the area of the posterior teeth.

4. _____ is having the jaws in a position that produces a centrally related occlusion.

5. A bar that joins the right and left quadrant framework of a partial denture is a(n) _____.

6. A(n) _____ is a dental laboratory device that simulates the movements of the mandible and the temporomandibular joint.

7. The surgical reduction and reshaping of the alveolar ridge is a(n)

   _____.

8. In _____ you use your fingers to contour a closer adaptation of the margins of an impression while still in the mouth.

9. A thin metal covering or cap placed over a prepared tooth is a(n)

   _____.

10. _____ means without teeth.

11. The _____ is a rigid, preformed shape used during the fitting of a full denture to temporarily represent the base of the denture.

12. The _____ is located on the lingual surface of the body of the mandible.

13. To trim or shape a denture to simulate normal tissue appearance is

_____.

14. The parts of a full or partial denture that extend from the teeth to the border of the denture are the _____.

15. A fold of tissue attaching the cheeks and lips to the upper and lower arches is the

_____.

16. The _____ is the metal skeleton of the removable partial denture.

17. Small, rounded, raised areas on the inner surface of the mandible are

_____.

18. _____ is the term for chewing.

19. The _____ is located on the facial surface of the mandible near the base of the ramus.

20. A(n) _____ is a prosthesis that replaces all of the teeth in one arch.

21. A temporary denture placed after the extraction of anterior teeth is a(n)

_____.

22. _____ is the sliding position of the mandible to the left or right of the centric position.

23. The _____ is built on the baseplate to register vertical

dimension and occlusal relationship of the mandibular and maxillary arches.

24. The _____ is a seal at the posterior of a full or partial denture that holds it in place.

25. Specific areas in the mouth where a removable prosthesis may rub or apply more pressure are the

_____.

26. _____ is the position of the mandible placed forward as related to the maxilla.

27. A(n) _____ is a removable prosthesis that replaces one or several teeth within the same arch.

28. _____ is the means of replacing the entire denture base material of an existing prosthesis.

29. _____ is the process of resurfacing the tissue side of a partial or full denture so that it fits more accurately.

30. _____ is the body's processes of removing existing bone or hard tissue structure.

31. A(n) _____ is a metal projection on or near the retainer of a partial denture.

32. The _____ is a device used to hold something in place such as the attachments or abutments of a removable prosthesis.

33. The portion of the mandible directly posterior to the last molar on each side is

the _____.

34. _____ is the position of the mandible posterior from the centric position as related to the maxilla.

MULTIPLE CHOICE

Complete each question by circling the best answer.

1. A removable prosthesis that replaces one or more teeth is called a:

   a. bridge.
   b. denture.
   c. partial.
   d. custom tray.

2. How can a person's occupation affect his or her choice in a removable prosthesis?

   a. Salary
   b. Appearance
   c. Confidence
   d. b and c

3. How can the presence of a new prosthesis affect the flow of saliva?

   a. Increase
   b. Decrease
   c. Change the texture
   d. No change

4. Why is an evenly contoured alveolar ridge so important to the way a removable prosthesis fits?

   a. Allows the patient to chew
   b. Gives a natural smile
   c. Provides a better fit
   d. a and c

5. What oral habits can affect the choice of a removable prosthesis?

   a. Clenching
   b. Grinding
   c. Mouth breathing
   d. All of the above

6. What is the metal skeleton of a partial called?

   a. Internal partial
   b. Framework
   c. Clasp
   d. Retainer

7. A retainer on a partial is also called a:

   a. connector.
   b. base.
   c. rest.
   d. clasp.

8. What component of a partial controls the way it is seated in the mouth?

   a. Connectors
   b. Base
   c. Rests
   d. Clasp

9. What impression material is commonly used when taking a final impression for a partial?

   a. Hydrocolloid
   b. Elastomeric
   c. Silicone
   d. Wax

10. What dental material does the laboratory technician set the teeth in for the try-in appointment for a denture?

    a. Alginate
    b. Plaster
    c. Stone
    d. Wax

11. The suction seal that is created between the denture and mouth is called the:

    a. post dam.
    b. base.
    c. border molding.
    d. reline.

12. How many teeth are in a full set of dentures?

    a. 8
    b. 16
    c. 28
    d. 32

13. What technique does the dentist use to modify the borders of an impression?

    a. Reline
    b. Tissue conditioning
    c. Articulate
    d. Border molding

14. What is a smile line?

    a. Space between the maxillary and mandibular teeth
    b. Amount of teeth showing when a patient smiles
    c. The shape of the teeth when a patient smiles
    d. How happy the patient is with the dentures

15. Which position of the jaw does the dentist measure when articulating a denture?

    a. Centric relation
    b. Protrusion
    c. Retrusion
    d. All of the above

16. When is an immediate denture most commonly used?

    a. After a root canal
    b. After extraction of anterior teeth
    c. After extraction of posterior teeth
    d. After periodontal surgery

17. What is the normal length of time for an immediate denture to be worn?

    a. A few days
    b. A few weeks
    c. A few months
    d. A year

18. How is an overdenture supported in the mouth?

    a. Teeth
    b. Tongue
    c. Oral mucosa
    d. a and c

19. The term for placing a new layer of resin over the tissue surface of a prosthesis is:

    a. border molding.
    b. relining.
    c. waxing.
    d. polishing.

20. Of the dental professions, who can legally repair a denture?

    a. Dentist
    b. Hygienist
    c. Laboratory technician
    d. a and c

CASE STUDY

A friend of the family comes to you for your advice. Her dentist has recommended that she have a partial made to replace teeth #18, #19, and #30, #31. She is confused as to the options that her dentist discussed with her, and she wants your opinion on what she should do.

1. What is your position on giving family and friends advice about their dental needs?
2. Why would a dentist recommend a partial rather than two separate bridges?
3. Why would a dentist recommend a partial rather than having the remaining teeth extracted and having a denture made?
4. Why would a dentist recommend a partial rather than having implants placed?
5. What is the role of the dental laboratory technician in making a partial?

53 | Dental Implants

SHORT ANSWER QUESTIONS

1. Discuss the indications and contraindications for dental implants.
2. Discuss the selection of patients to receive dental implants.
3. Identify the different types of dental implants.
4. Describe the surgical procedures for implantation.
5. Describe the home care procedures and follow-up visits required after receiving dental implants.

FILL IN THE BLANK

Select the best term from the list below and complete the following statements.

Circumoral
Endosteal
Implant
Osseointegration
Peri-implant tissue
Subperiosteal
Surgical stent
Titanium
Transosteal

1. An implant that is inserted through the inferior border of the mandible is a(n)

   _____.

2. An implant that is surgically embedded into the bone is a(n) _____.

3. _____ is the attachment of healthy bone to a dental implant.

4. _____ means surrounding the mouth.

5. A(n) _____ is a type of implant with a metal frame placed under the periosteum, but on top of the bone.

6. The _____ is gingival sulcus surrounding the implant.

7. A clear acrylic template that is placed over the alveolar ridge to help locate the proper placement for dental implants is a(n)

   _____.

8. A(n) _____ is artificial teeth that are attached to anchors that have been surgically embedded into the bone or surrounding structures.

9. _____ is a type of metal used for implants.

MULTIPLE CHOICE

Complete each question by circling the best answer.

1. Which dental specialist has training in dental implants?

   a. Oral and maxillofacial surgeon
   b. Periodontist
   c. Prosthodontist
   d. All of the above

2. What is the success rate for dental implants?

   a. 50%
   b. 70%
   c. 90%
   d. 100%

3. How long can dental implants last?

   a. 5 to 10 years
   b. 10 to 20 years
   c. 20 to 30 years
   d. A lifetime

4. Compared to fixed prosthodontics, what is the financial investment for an implant?

   a. Greater than fixed prosthodontics
   b. Less than fixed prosthodontics
   c. About the same cost
   d. Insurance will cover the difference

5. How long could an implant procedure take from beginning to the final?

   a. 2 weeks
   b. 6 weeks
   c. 9 months
   d. 1 year

6. Which radiograph is used by the dentist for the evaluation of a patient for implants?

   a. Panoramic
   b. Cephalometric
   c. Tomogram
   d. All of the above

7. How is a surgical stent used during implant surgery?

   a. To hold the tissue in place
   b. To guide placement of the implant
   c. To maintain the teeth in an upright position
   d. To assist in the healing process

8. What material is an implant made from?

   a. Bone graft
   b. Stainless steel
   c. Titanium
   d. Enamel

9. *Osseo* means:

   a. implant.
   b. tissue.
   c. splint.
   d. bone.

10. What component of the endosteal implant attaches to the artificial tooth or teeth?

    a. Abutment post
    b. Cylinder
    c. Stent
    d. a and b

11. When would a subperiosteal implant be recommended for use?

    a. Maxillary anterior
    b. Mandibular full denture
    c. Mandibular anterior
    d. Maxillary full denture

12. Why is plaque and calculus easier to remove from implants than from natural teeth?

    a. Implants have a rough surface
    b. Implants have a natural cleansing cover
    c. Implants have a smooth surface
    d. Implants have fluoride embedded in the teeth

13. Which is an example of a cleaning accessory used for implants?

    a. Toothbrush
    b. Clasp brush
    c. Interproximal brush
    d. All of the above

CASE STUDY

Your patient is considering implants. However, he sees two drawbacks to having the procedure. One is the cost, and the other is that it will take so long for the procedure to be completed.

1. Are there any contraindications that should be reviewed with a patient before starting?
2. Explain why the process of implants takes so long, and the importance of not rushing through.
3. What role does infection control play in the procedure of implants?
4. What options could the patient be made aware of in regards to financial assistance for having implants?
5. Describe the most important home care advice that this patient should receive about implants.

54 | Endodontics

SHORT ANSWER QUESTIONS

1. List the diagnostic testing procedures performed for endodontic diagnosis.
2. List the conclusions of the subjective and objective tests in endodontic diagnosis.
3. Describe diagnostic conclusions for endodontic therapy.
4. List the types of endodontic procedures.
5. Discuss the medicaments and dental materials used in endodontics.
6. Give an overview of root canal therapy.
7. Describe surgical endodontics and how it affects treatment.

FILL IN THE BLANK

Select the best term from the list below and complete the following statements.

Abscess
Acute
Apical curettage
Apicoectomy
Chronic
Control tooth
Débridement
Endodontist
Gutta percha
Hemisection
Indirect pulp cap
Irreversible pulpitis
Nonvital
Obturate
Palpitation
Percussion
Perforation
Periradicular
Pulp cap
Pulpectomy
Pulpitis
Pulpotomy
Retrograde restoration
Reversible pulpitis
Root amputation
Root canal therapy

1. _____ is the surgical removal of infectious material surrounding the apex of a root.

2. A(n) _____ is the surgical removal of the apical portion of the tooth through a surgical opening made in the overlying bone and gingival tissues.

3. Something that persists over a long period of time is said to be

_____.

4. A(n) _____ is a healthy tooth used as a standard to compare questionable teeth of similar size and structure during pulp vitality testing.

5. _____ is a localized area of pus originating from an infection.

6. An immediate response is to be

_____.

7. _____ is when the pulp is incapable of healing and will require a root canal.

8. _____ is the examination technique that involves tapping on the incisal or occlusal surface of a tooth to determine vitality.

9. _____ is a plastic type of filling material used in endodontics.

10. The surgical separation of a multirooted tooth through the furcation area is a(n)

_____.

11. A(n) _____ is the placement of a medicament over a partially exposed pulp.

12. _____ means not living.

13. _____ is completed to remove or clean out the pulpal canal.

14. _____ is the examination technique of the soft tissues with the examiner's hand or fingertips.

15. A(n) _____ is the removal of one or more roots without removing the crown of the tooth.

16. _____ is the procedure in the removal of the dental pulp and filling the canal with material.

17. _____ is the process of filling a root canal.

18. A(n) _____ is the application of a material to a cavity preparation that has exposed or nearly exposed the dental pulp.

19. To break through and extend beyond the apex of the root is _____.

20. Nerves, blood vessels, and tissue that surround the root of a tooth are called _____.

21. A(n) _____ is the complete removal of a vital pulp from a tooth.

22. A(n) _____ is the removal of the coronal portion of a vital pulp from a tooth.

23. _____ is the inflammation of the dental pulp.

24. A small restoration placed at the apex of a root is a(n) _____.

25. A dentist who specializes with the prevention, diagnosis, and treatment of the dental pulp and periradicular tissues is a(n) _____.

26. _____ is when there is inflammation of the dental pulp, but the pulp may be able to be saved.

MULTIPLE CHOICE

Complete each question by circling the best answer.

1. What are periradicular tissues?
   a. Pulp tissue
   b. Tissue that surrounds the root of the tooth
   c. Tissue that surrounds the crown of the tooth
   d. Buccal mucosa

2. Which specialist performs root canal therapy?
   a. Prosthodontist
   b. Implantologist
   c. Endodontist
   d. Periodontist

3. What will result if bacteria reach the nerves and blood vessels of a tooth?
   a. Abscess
   b. Decay
   c. Tumor
   d. Calculus

4. Is pain a subjective or objective component of a diagnosis?
   a. Subjective
   b. Objective
   c. Neither
   d. Both

5. Tooth #5 is being tested for possible endodontic treatment. What tooth would be used as a control tooth?
   a. #6
   b. #9
   c. #12
   d. #15

6. When the dentist taps on a tooth, what diagnostic test is being performed?
   a. Mobility
   b. Heat
   c. Palpitation
   d. Percussion

7. What type of radiograph is taken through the course of root canal therapy?
   a. Full mouth series
   b. Bite-wing
   c. Periapical
   d. Panorex

8. What diagnosis is given when pulp tissues become inflamed?

    a. Pulpitis
    b. Pulpotomy
    c. Pulpectomy
    d. Abscess

9. Another term for *necrotic* is:

    a. living.
    b. dead.
    c. nonvital.
    d. b and c

10. What dental material is used for pulp capping?

    a. Alginate
    b. Zinc phosphate
    c. Calcium hydroxide
    d. Glass ionomer

11. How much of a pulp is removed in a pulpotomy?

    a. Coronal portion
    b. Root portion
    c. Complete pulp
    d. Just the infected portion

12. What instrument has tiny projections and is used to remove pulp tissue?

    a. File
    b. Broach
    c. Reamer
    d. Pesso file

13. How are endodontic files used?

    a. Slow-speed handpiece
    b. High-speed handpiece
    c. By hand manipulation
    d. Syringe

14. What type of file is best suited for canal enlargement?

    a. Broach
    b. Reamer
    c. Pesso file
    d. Hedstom file

15. The rubber stop is placed on a file to:

    a. prevent perforation.
    b. maintain the correct measurement of the canal.
    c. identify the file.
    d. a and b

16. *Obturate* means to:

    a. open a pulpal canal.
    b. examine a pulpal canal.
    c. fill a pulpal canal.
    d. surgically remove the pulpal canal.

17. What is most commonly used as an irrigation solution during root canal therapy?

    a. Water from the air-water syringe
    b. Diluted sodium hypochlorite
    c. Concentrated sodium hypochlorite
    d. Phosphoric acid

18. What material is used for obturation of a canal?

    a. Amalgam
    b. Composite
    c. Gutta percha
    d. IRM

19. What type of moisture control is recommended for root canal therapy?

    a. Cotton pellets
    b. Cotton rolls
    c. Dry angles
    d. Dental dam

20. What surface of an anterior tooth does the dentist enter when performing root canal therapy?

    a. Lingual
    b. Facial
    c. Mesial
    d. Incisal

21. What is the success rate of root canal therapy?

    a. 60% to 65%
    b. 70% to 75%
    c. 80% to 85%
    d. 90% to 95%

22. What surgical procedure involves the removal of the apex of a root?

    a. Hemisection
    b. Apicoectomy
    c. Forceps extraction
    d. Pulpotomy

CASE STUDY

John Allen is being seen today for root canal therapy on tooth #20. This is Mr. Allen's first time to the endodontist, and he seems to be in quite a bit of pain and discomfort.

1. How would Mr. Allen have known to come to an endodontist for dental treatment?
2. What type of tooth is #20, and how many canals could possibly be affected?
3. What type of diagnostic testing has the dentist completed to determine that the tooth requires endodontic treatment?
4. What tooth is used as the control tooth during diagnostic evaluation, and why is a control tooth used?
5. What type of pain control would the endodontist use to help alleviate stress as well as discomfort during the procedure for Mr. Allen?

55 | Periodontics

SHORT ANSWER QUESTIONS

1. Describe the role of the dental assistant in a periodontal practice.
2. Explain the procedures necessary for a comprehensive periodontal examination.
3. Describe the instruments used in periodontal therapy.
4. Give the indications for placement of periodontal surgical dressings, and describe the technique for proper placement.
5. Describe systemic conditions that can influence periodontal treatment.
6. Describe the role of radiographs in periodontal treatment.
7. Describe the indications and contraindications for use of the ultrasonic scaler.
8. Describe the types of nonsurgical periodontal therapy.
9. Describe the types of surgical periodontal therapy.

FILL IN THE BLANK

Select the best term from the list below and complete the following statements.

Bleeding index
Gingivectomy
Gingivoplasty
Laser beam
Mobility
Osseous surgery
Ostectomy
Osteoplasty
Periodontal dressing
Periodontal explorers
Periodontal pockets
Pcriodontics
Periodontist
Ultrasonic scaler

1. The dental specialty that deals with the diagnosis and treatment of diseases of the

   supporting tissues is _____.

2. A(n) _____ is a dentist with advanced education in the specialty of periodontics.

3. _____ are a deepening of the gingival sulcus beyond normal, resulting from periodontal disease.

4. A surgical dressing that is applied to the surgical site for protection, similar to a

   bandage, is a(n) _____.

5. Movement of the tooth in its socket is

   called _____.

6. The _____ is a method of scoring the amount of bleeding present.

7. _____ are a type of explorer that is thin, fine, and easily adapted around root surfaces.

8. A(n) _____ is a device used for rapid calculus removal that operates on high-frequency sound waves.

9. _____ is performed to remove defects in bone.

10. _____ is the surgical removal of diseased gingival tissues.

11. A type of surgery in which gingival tissues are reshaped and contoured is

    _____.

12. _____ is a type of surgery in which bone is added, contoured, and reshaped.

13. _____ is a type of surgery involving the removal of bone.

14. A highly concentrated beam of light is a

    _____.

MULTIPLE CHOICE

Complete each question by circling the best answer.

1. How do patients most often seek periodontal care?

   a. Prescription by their general dentist
   b. Referral by their general dentist
   c. Referral by another specialist
   d. Referral by their insurance company

2. What information is included in periodontal charting?

   a. Pocket readings
   b. Furcations
   c. Tooth mobility
   d. All of the above

3. Should teeth have any mobility?

   a. No
   b. Depends on the teeth
   c. A slight amount
   d. Yes

4. What is the depth of a normal sulcus?

   a. 1 to 3 mm
   b. 2 to 4 mm
   c. 3 to 5 mm
   d. 4 to 6 mm

5. What unit of measurement is used on the periodontal probe?

   a. Centimeters
   b. Millimeters
   c. Inches
   d. Milligrams

6. What type of radiograph is especially useful in periodontics?

   a. Panoramic
   b. Occlusal
   c. Bite-wing
   d. Periapical

7. Which instrument is used to remove calculus from supragingival surfaces?

   a. Spoon excavator
   b. Scaler
   c. Explorer
   d. Curette

8. Which type of instrument is used to remove calculus from subgingival surfaces?

   a. Spoon excavator
   b. Scaler
   c. Explorer
   d. Curette

9. What is the purpose of explorers in periodontal treatment?

   a. Detect pathology
   b. Provide tactile information
   c. Examine the occlusion
   d. Apply sealants

10. Which type of curette has two cutting edges?

    a. Universal
    b. Kirkland
    c. Gracey
    d. Sickle

11. What is the purpose of a periodontal pocket marker?

    a. Carry items to and from the mouth
    b. To make bleeding points in the gingival tissue
    c. Measure the sulcus
    d. Remove calculus from the sulcus

12. How do ultrasonic scalers work?

    a. Water pressure
    b. Air pressure
    c. Sound waves
    d. Rpm

13. What oral conditions would contraindicate the use of an ultrasonic scaler?

    a. Patients with demineralization
    b. Narrow periodontal pockets
    c. Exposed dentin
    d. All of the above

14. Should an ultrasonic scaler be used on a patient with a communicable disease?

    a. Yes
    b. No
    c. It does not matter

15. What is the more common term for a dental prophylaxis?

    a. Prophy
    b. Sealants
    c. Scaling
    d. Treatment

16. Who can perform a dental prophylaxis?

    a. Dentist
    b. Dental assistant
    c. Dental hygienist
    d. a and c

17. Which is a surgical periodontal treatment?

    a. Scaling
    b. Root planing
    c. Gingivectomy
    d. Gingival curettage

18. What drug is often used for to treat periodontitis, juvenile periodontitis, and rapidly destructive periodontitis?

    a. Fluoride
    b. Tetracycline
    c. Ibuprofen
    d. Acetaminophen

1. What type of dental professional would complete this procedure?
2. What is another name for incisional periodontal surgery?
3. In setting up the surgical tray, what additional items will be retrieved for the excision?
4. In closing this flap, what would the surgeon most commonly use?
5. To protect the surgical site and promote healing, what will you prepare for placement? Where would this be placed?

CASE STUDY

You will be assisting Dr. Lanier this morning with an incisional periodontal surgery. Dr. Lanier has noted in the patient record that teeth #23 through #26 do not have adequate tissue coverage, and he will need to move the flap of tissue into position to cover more tooth structure.

56 | Oral and Maxillofacial Surgery

SHORT ANSWER QUESTIONS

1. Define the specialty of oral and maxillofacial surgery.
2. Discuss the role of an oral surgery assistant.
3. State the importance of the chain of asepsis during a surgical procedure.
4. Describe the surgical procedures commonly performed in a general practice.
5. Describe the type of postoperative care given to a patient after a surgical procedure.
6. Discuss the possible complications from surgery.

FILL IN THE BLANK

Select the best term from the list below and complete the following statements.

Alveoplasty
Bone file
Chisel
Donning
Elevator
Excisional biopsy
Forceps
Gurney
Hard-tissue impaction
Hemostat
Impacted tooth
Incisional biopsy
Mallet
Needle holder
Oral and maxillofacial surgeon
Oral and maxillofacial surgery
Outpatient
Retractor
Rongeur
Scalpel
Soft tissue impaction
Surgical curette

1. The _____ is a surgical instrument used for cutting or severing a tooth and bone structure.

2. A surgical instrument used to reflect and retract the periodontal ligament and periosteum is the _____.

3. A(n) _____ is a mobile table to transport patients.

4. A(n) _____ is a tooth that is partial to fully covered by bone and gingival tissue.

5. An instrument used to hold or grasp items is a(n) _____.

6. A(n) _____ is a surgical instrument used to remove tissue from the tooth socket.

7. _____ is the surgical reduction and reshaping of the alveolar ridge.

8. A surgical instrument used to smooth rough edges of bone structure is a(n) _____.

9. A(n) _____ is a tooth that is partially to fully covered by gingival tissue.

10. A(n) _____ is the procedure to cut and examine questionable tissue from its site.

11. The _____ is an instrument used to hold the suture needle.

12. A surgical instrument used to grasp and hold on to teeth for their removal is _____.

13. _____ is the act of placing an item on, such as gloves.

14. A tooth that has not erupted is termed a(n) _____.

15. A(n) _____ is a section of a questionable lesion that is removed for evaluation.

16. A(n) _____ is a hammerlike instrument, used along with a chisel to section teeth or bone.

17. A(n) _____ is a surgical knife.

18. A(n) _____ is a dentist that has specialized in surgeries of the head and neck region.

19. _____ is the specialty of dentistry that specializes in the treatment of head and neck.

20. A patient who is seen and treated by a doctor and then sent home for recovery is considered a(n) _____.

21. _____ is an instrument used to hold back soft tissue.

22. The _____ is a surgical instrument used to cut and trim the alveolar bone.

MULTIPLE CHOICE

Complete each question by circling the best answer.

1. The surgical procedure that a general dentist most commonly performs is:
   a. forceps extraction.
   b. removal of impacted teeth.
   c. reconstructive surgery.
   d. biopsy.

2. How can a dental assistant further his or her profession as a surgical assistant?
   a. Obtain a dental hygiene degree
   b. Obtain a nursing degree
   c. Obtain continuing education in oral and maxillofacial surgery
   d. Obtain a dental degree

3. In what type of settings are oral surgery procedures completed?
   a. Dental office
   b. Outpatient clinic
   c. Hospital
   d. All of the above

4. Most oral and maxillofacial surgeries are considered to be:
   a. major surgery.
   b. minor surgery.
   c. dental procedure.
   d. medical procedure.

5. What does the periosteal elevator reflect and retract?
   a. Gingival tissue
   b. Tooth
   c. Periosteum
   d. Lips

6. Give the number assigned to the universal forceps for the maxillary and mandibular molars.
   a. 70 / 72
   b. 89 / 98
   c. 110 / 112
   d. 150 / 151

7. What surgical instrument resembles a spoon excavator?
   a. Rongeur
   b. Surgical curette
   c. Elevator
   d. Scalpel

8. What surgical instrument is used to trim and shape bone?
   a. Rongeur
   b. Surgical curette
   c. Elevator
   d. Scalpel

9. When setting up the chisel, what additional surgical instrument must be set out?
   a. Elevator
   b. Scalpel
   c. Mallet
   d. Hemostat

10. What equipment is used to perform a surgical scrub?

    a. Orange stick
    b. Antimicrobial soap
    c. Scrub brush
    d. All of the above

11. What does the term *donning* mean?

    a. Taking off
    b. Placing on
    c. Procedure
    d. Prior to

12. What procedure is completed directly after the removal of multiple teeth?

    a. Implants
    b. Sutures
    c. Alveoplasty
    d. Alveolitis

13. When a tooth is directly under gingival tissue, it is said to be:

    a. anklyosed.
    b. soft-tissue impacted.
    c. exposed.
    d. hard-tissue impacted.

14. What type of biopsy is completed when a surface lesion is scraped to attain cells?

    a. Incisional biopsy
    b. Excisional biopsy
    c. Exfoliative biopsy
    d. Surgical biopsy

15. The term *suture* refers to:

    a. impaction.
    b. stitching.
    c. control of bleeding.
    d. multiple extractions.

16. Of the suture types listed, which is an absorbable suture material?

    a. Silk
    b. Polyester
    c. Nylon
    d. Catgut

17. What is the approximate time frame for removing nonabsorbable sutures?

    a. 1 to 3 days
    b. 4 to 6 days
    c. 5 to 7 days
    d. 12 to 14 days

18. How long should a pressure pack remain on a surgical site to control bleeding?

    a. 30 minutes
    b. 2 to 3 hours
    c. 12 hours
    d. 24 hours

19. What analgesic may be prescribed for swelling?

    a. Antibiotic
    b. Ibuprofen
    c. Aspirin
    d. Codeine

20. What should a patient place to control swelling?

    a. Gauze pack
    b. Hydrocolloid
    c. Cold pack
    d. Heat pack

CASE STUDY

Katie Samuels is a patient of referral and is calling due to extreme pain in her lower right jaw. The business assistant pulls her record and reviews that Katie had teeth #17 and #32 surgically removed 3 days ago. The teeth had been impacted, but the notes by the surgeon indicated that the procedure went well. Katie is scheduled to come in a week for a check and suture removal.

1. Why would this patient be referred to a specialist for having these teeth extracted?
2. Give a possible diagnosis for Katie's pain.
3. What could have possibly caused this problem? If the diagnosis is correct, what could be done to alleviate Katie's pain?
4. Can the patient wait until her scheduled check to be seen? If not, when should the patient be seen?

57 | Pediatric Dentistry

SHORT ANSWER QUESTIONS

1. Describe the appearance and setting of a pediatric dental office.
2. Discuss the pediatric patient and the stages experienced by children from birth through adolescence.
3. Discuss the specific behavior techniques that work as a positive reinforcement in the treatment of children.
4. Describe why children and adults with special needs are treated in a pediatric practice.
5. List the steps involved in the diagnosis and treatment planning of a pediatric patient.
6. Discuss the importance of preventive dentistry in pediatrics.
7. Describe the clinical procedures for the pediatric patient compared with the treatment of permanent teeth.

FILL IN THE BLANK

Select the best term from the list below and complete the following statements.

Analogy
Athetosis
Autonomy
Avulsed
Cerebral palsy
Chronological age
Contoured
Crossbite
Down syndrome
Emotional age
Extrusion
Festooned
Frankyl scale
Intrusion
Luxation
Mental age
Mental retardation
Neural
Open bay
Papoose board
Pediatric dentistry
Postnatal
Pulpotomy
Prenatal

Spasticity
T-band

1. _____ is a neural disorder caused by brain damage.

2. A child's actual age is his or her

_____.

3. _____ is to shape or conform an object.

4. A(n) _____ is a comparison with something that is similar.

5. _____ is the process of being independent.

6. An object or item that is torn away or dislodged by force is said to be

_____.

7. A(n) _____ is where the facial aspects of the maxillary teeth are located lingual to the mandibular teeth.

8. _____ is a disorder that is caused by a chromosome defect.

9. _____ is involuntary movement of the body, face, arms, and legs.

10. The _____ describes the child's level of emotional maturity.

11. _____ is when teeth are displaced out of the socket as a result of an injury.

12. When teeth are displaced into the socket as a result of an injury, they are said to be _____.

13. _____ is an exaggerated movement by the arms and legs.

14. The _____ is a type of matrix band used for primary teeth.

15. _____ means to dislocate.

16. A child's _____ determines his or her level of intellectual capacity and development.

17. When an object is trimmed or shaped it is said to be _____.

18. The _____ is a scale designed to evaluate behavior.

19. The specialty of dentistry concerned with the infant through adolescent and the special-needs patient is _____.

20. _____ means after birth.

21. _____ is a disorder in which an individual's intelligence is underdeveloped.

22. Another term for the brain is the _____.

23. _____ is an open concept of office design used in pediatric dental practices.

24. A(n) _____ is a type of restraining device to hold hands, arms, and legs still.

25. A(n) _____ is a dental procedure that removes the coronal portion of the dental pulp.

26. _____ means before birth.

MULTIPLE CHOICE

Complete each question by circling the best answer.

1. At what age would a person most likely stop going to a pediatric dentist?

   a. 12
   b. 14
   c. 17
   d. 21

2. What is unique about the treatment areas of a pediatric practice?

   a. Dental chairs are close together
   b. More than one dentist can use a treatment area
   c. The open bay concept
   d. Chair for the parent to sit in

3. Describe the types of patients seen in a pediatric practice.

   a. Healthy adolescents
   b. Special-needs children
   c. Special-needs adults
   d. All of the above

4. What are you describing about a child who is 10 years old but acts as if he is 8?

   a. His chronological age
   b. His emotional age
   c. His physical age
   d. His size

5. At what stage of a child's life does he or she first want control and structure of the environment?

   a. 1 to 3 years of age
   b. 3 to 5 years of age
   c. 6 to 9 years of age
   d. 9 to 12 years of age

6. How would Dr. Frankyl describe a positive child?

   a. Accepts treatment
   b. Willing to comply
   c. Follows directions
   d. All of the above

7. When would a papoose board be used?

   a. For a sedated young child
   b. For an extraction on a 12-year-old
   c. In the placement of sealants
   d. For a fluoride treatment

8. What limits children when they are mentally challenged?

   a. Physical ability
   b. Speech
   c. IQ
   d. b and c

9. Another name for Down syndrome is:

   a. trisomy 21.
   b. mental retardation.
   c. cerebral palsy.
   d. learning disorder.

10. At what age is it common for a person to be afflicted with cerebral palsy?

    a. Young child
    b. Preteen
    c. Young adult
    d. a and c

11. At what age should a child first see a dentist for a regular exam?

    a. 2
    b. 4
    c. 6
    d. 8

12. If a patient has a high risk of decay, how often should radiographs be taken?

    a. Monthly
    b. Every 6 months
    c. Once a year
    d. Before the tooth is restored

13. How is fluoride varnish used in the United States?

    a. As a fluoride rinse
    b. As prescription fluoride
    c. As a desensitizer
    d. As a liner

14. What procedure is recommended for children to protect the pits and fissures of posterior teeth?

    a. Pulpotomy
    b. Fluoride rinse
    c. Coronal polishing
    d. Sealants

15. At what phase of orthodontics will a pediatric dentist intercede to get a patient to stop sucking his or her thumb?

    a. Interceptive
    b. Preventive
    c. Corrective
    d. Elective

16. If you are a competitive swimmer, should you wear a mouth guard?

    a. No
    b. Yes

17. What types of matrices are used on primary teeth?

    a. Metal contoured
    b. T-band
    c. Spot welded
    d. b and c

18. What endodontic procedure is performed on primary teeth?

    a. Apicoectomy
    b. Pulpectomy
    c. Pulpotomy
    d. Implant

19. Would a child be referred to a prosthodontist for placement of a stainless steel crown?

    a. Yes
    b. No

20. What teeth are most frequently injured in the mouth?

    a. Mandibular anterior
    b. Mandibular posterior
    c. Maxillary anterior
    d. Maxillary posterior

21. When a tooth is avulsed, it has:

    a. been fractured.
    b. come out.
    c. pushed back into the socket.
    d. become loose.

22. How will a dentist stabilize a tooth after an injury?

    a. Temporary splint
    b. Thermoplastic resin tray
    c. Wax
    d. Sutures

23. Who in the dental office is legally required to report child abuse?

    a. Dental assistant
    b. Business assistant
    c. Dental hygienist
    d. Dentist

24. What could be a possible sign of child abuse?

    a. Chipped or fractured teeth
    b. Bruises
    c. Scars on the lips or tongue
    d. All of the above

25. What organization should be contacted if someone suspects child abuse?

    a. American Dental Association
    b. Child protective services of the public health department
    c. Local hospital
    d. Pediatric Dental Association

CASE STUDY

Ashley is a 12-year-old patient of the practice and is being seen as an emergency patient. While playing intramural basketball, Ashley was hit in the face, which knocked her maxillary central incisors back into the socket.

1. If your schedule is filled for the day, when should the business assistant have Ashley come in for an emergency visit?
2. What type of examination techniques could be used to enable the dentist to make a correct diagnosis of the complexity of the teeth's damage?
3. What is the diagnosis if person's teeth are knocked inward?
4. Are these Ashley's primary or permanent central incisors?
5. What form of treatment would be provided for Ashley today?

58 | Coronal Polishing

SHORT ANSWER QUESTIONS

1. Explain the difference between a prophylaxis and coronal polishing.
2. Explain the indications and contraindications for a coronal polish.
3. Name and describe the types of extrinsic stains.
4. Name and describe the two categories of intrinsic stains.
5. Describe four types of abrasives used for polishing the teeth.

FILL IN THE BLANK

Select the best term from the list below and complete the following statements.

Calculus
Clinical crown
Extrinsic stain
Fulcrum
Intrinsic stain
Oral prophylaxis
Rubber cup polishing

1. _____ is a hard, mineralized deposit attached to the teeth.

2. A(n) _____ is the complete removal of calculus, debris, stains, and plaque from the teeth.

3. The portion of the tooth that is visible in the oral cavity is the _____.

4. Stains that occur within the tooth structure and may not be removed by polishing are _____.

5. Stains that occur on the external surfaces of the teeth and may be removed by polishing are _____.

6. The _____ is a position that provides stability for the operator.

7. _____ is a technique used to remove plaque and stains from the coronal surfaces of the teeth.

MULTIPLE CHOICE

Complete each question by circling the best answer.

1. The purpose of coronal polishing is:

   a. to remove calculus.
   b. to remove stains and plaque.
   c. to prepare teeth for a restoration.
   d. to remove inflamed gingiva.

2. An oral prophylaxis includes:

   a. fluoride treatment.
   b. removal of calculus and debris.
   c. examination.
   d. removal of decay.

3. What is the purpose of selective polishing?

   a. To polish teeth that are only visible
   b. To polish the occlusal surfaces of the teeth
   c. To polish only the teeth that have stains
   d. To polish the facial surfaces of teeth

4. A stain that may be removed from the surfaces of the teeth is called a(n):

   a. extrinsic stain.
   b. natural stain.
   c. intrinsic stain.
   d. infected stain.

5. A stain that cannot be removed from the surfaces of the teeth is called a(n):

   a. extrinsic stain.
   b. natural stain.
   c. intrinsic stain.
   d. infected stain.

6. Which is the most common technique for stain removal?

   a. Scaler
   b. Toothbrush
   c. Floss
   d. Rubber cup polishing

7. Which grasp is used to hold the handpiece?

   a. Reverse palm grasp
   b. Pen grasp
   c. Thumb-to-nose grasp
   d. Palm grasp

8. What is the purpose of a fulcrum?

   a. To provide pressure to the fingers
   b. To provide better retraction
   c. To provide stability to the hand
   d. To provide movement for the arm

9. What precaution should be taken when using a bristle brush?

   a. Do not allow the brush to get dry
   b. Not to traumatize the tissue
   c. Not to wear away the enamel
   d. Not to use on occlusal surfaces

10. The polishing stroke should be in which direction?

    a. Toward the incisal
    b. Toward the gingiva
    c. Toward the occlusal
    d. a and c

11. What damage can result from using the prophy angle at a high speed?

    a. Cause frictional heat
    b. Remove dentin
    c. Cool the tooth
    d. Etch enamel

12. How should the patient's head be positioned for access to the maxillary and mandibular anteriors?

    a. Chin downward
    b. Head turned to the right
    c. Chin upward
    d. Head turned to the left

CASE STUDY

You are a preventive clinical assistant in a very busy pediatric office. A daily schedule for a preventive assistant usually includes seeing 8 to 10 patients daily. The patients who are scheduled for you include new patient appointments, emergencies, and recall patients.

1. Describe the specific procedures for which you would be responsible for a recall patient.
2. Is it possible for a pediatric practice not to have a dental hygienist? If so, how?
3. Because you work with children, what contraindications would keep you from completing a coronal polishing on a patient?
4. During the evaluation of a recall patient, you notice calculus located on the lingual surfaces of the lower anteriors. How would this calculus be removed, and who will remove it?
5. Would calculus be removed before the coronal polishing or after?

59 | Dental Sealants

SHORT ANSWER QUESTIONS

1. Describe the purpose of dental sealants.
2. Give the clinical indications for dental sealants.
3. Discuss the rationale for filled and unfilled sealant materials.
4. Describe the two types of polymerization.
5. Give the steps in the application of dental sealants.
6. Describe the safety steps necessary for patient and operator during sealant placement.
7. Explain the most important factor in sealant retention.

FILL IN THE BLANK

Select the best term from the list below and complete the following statements.

Acrylate
Dental sealant
Filled resin
Light-cured
Microleakage
Polymerization
Sealant retention
Self-cured
Unfilled resin

1. Resin material applied to the pits and fissures of the teeth is _____.

2. _____ is a process of changing a simple chemical into another substance containing the same elements.

3. A type of material that is polymerized by chemical reactions is _____.

4. A type of material that is polymerized by a curing light is _____.

5. _____ is a sealant material that contains filler particles.

6. _____ is a sealant material that does not contain filler particles.

7. _____ is a microscopic leakage at the interface of the tooth structure and the sealant or restoration.

8. _____ is a salt or ester of acrylic acid.

9. The sealant firmly adheres to the tooth surface because of _____.

MULTIPLE CHOICE

Complete each question by circling the best answer.

1. The purpose of dental sealants is to:

   a. prevent decay from spreading
   b. prevent decay from pits and fissures of teeth
   c. promote good oral health
   d. prevent decay from interproximal spaces

2. Why are pits and fissures susceptible to caries?

   a. Saliva pools in these areas
   b. Fluoride cannot reach this area
   c. Hard to evaluate on a radiograph
   d. Bacteria cannot be removed from these areas

3. Are sealants the only preventive measure used?

   a. Yes
   b. No

4. What are the ways for sealant materials to harden?

   a. Polymerization
   b. Light-cure
   c. Self-cure
   d. All of the above

5. Why is clear sealant material less desirable?

   a. Less attractive
   b. Difficult to evaluate
   c. Does not match tooth color
   d. Is contraindicated with dental restorations

6. What difference is there in filled and unfilled sealants in regards to retention rates?

   a. No difference
   b. Filled is much stronger
   c. Unfilled lasts longer
   d. Filler is weaker

7. Sealants are placed:

   a. in pits and fissures.
   b. on cingulums.
   c. in groves.
   d. on marginal ridges.

8. What is the range of shelf life of sealant materials?

   a. 3 to 6 months
   b. 6 to 12 months
   c. 18 to 36 months
   d. Indefinitely

9. What are patient safety precautions to keep in mind when placing sealants?

   a. Keep the etchant off the soft tissue
   b. Only use after patient has been anesthetized
   c. Have patient wear eyewear
   d. a and c

10. What determines the effectiveness of dental sealants?

   a. Polymerization
   b. Retention
   c. Cementation
   d. Occlusion

CASE STUDY

Cindy Evans is 8 years old and is scheduled to have sealants placed on all of her molars today. Dr. Allen is running behind and has told you to go ahead with the placement, and to call him if you have any questions.

1. What must Dr. Allen complete before you can begin the procedure?
2. How many teeth will receive sealants today?
3. Because you are working on your own, what type of moisture control will you use?
4. Describe your plan of preparation and placement of sealants.
5. After placement, Cindy complains of not being able to close her teeth. What is wrong, and how can you fix it?

60 | Orthodontics

SHORT ANSWER QUESTIONS

1. Describe the environment of an orthodontic practice.
2. Describe the types of malocclusion.
3. Discuss corrective orthodontics and what type of treatment is involved.
4. List the types of diagnostic records used to assess orthodontic problems.
5. Describe the components of the fixed appliance.
6. Describe the use and function of headgear.
7. Describe how you would convey the importance of dietary and good oral hygiene habits in the treatment of orthodontics.

FILL IN THE BLANK

Select the best term from the list below and complete the following statements.

Arch wire
Auxiliary
Band
Braces
Bracket
Cephalometric
Crossbite
Crowding
Dentofacial
Distoclusion
Fetal molding
Headgear
Ligature tie
Malocclusion
Mesioclusion
Occlusion
Open bite
Orthodontics
Overbite
Overjet
Positioner
Retainer
Separator

1. A(n) _____ is a stainless steel ring cemented to molars to hold the arch wire and additional auxiliaries for orthodontics.

2. Structures that include the teeth, jaws, and surrounding facial bones are the _____ structures.

3. Another term for a fixed orthodontic appliance is _____.

4. A(n) _____ is a small device bonded to teeth to hold the arch wire to the teeth.

5. _____ occurs when teeth are not aligned properly within the arch.

6. A(n) _____ wire is used to hold the arch wire in place.

7. Attachments that are on brackets and bands to hold arch wires and elastics are a(n) _____.

8. A(n) _____ is a shaped metal wire that provides force when guiding teeth in movement for orthodontics.

9. A(n) _____ is a device made from wire or elastic used to separate molars before fitting and placement of orthodontic bands.

10. Any occlusion that is deviated from a class I normal occlusion is called _____.

11. _____ is a another term for class III malocclusion.

12. An extraoral radiograph of the bones and tissues of the head is a(n) _____.

13. A(n) _____ is the malalignment of teeth, where the

maxillary teeth are located lingual to the mandibular teeth.

14. _____ is another term used for class II malocclusion.

15. An external orthodontic appliance used to control growth and tooth movement is

_____.

16. An appliance used for maintaining the positions of the teeth and jaws after orthodontic treatment is a(n)

_____.

17. An excessive protrusion of the maxillary

incisors is a(n) _____.

18. A lack of vertical overlap of the maxillary incisors that creates an opening of the

anterior teeth is a(n) _____.

19. _____ is the specialty of dentistry designed to prevent, intercept, and correct skeletal and dental problems.

20. A person's _____ is the way the maxillary and mandibular teeth come together.

21. A(n) _____ is a type of appliance used to retain teeth in their desired position.

22. An increased vertical overlap of the

maxillary incisors is a(n) _____.

23. _____ can occur when pressure is applied to the jaw, causing a distortion.

MULTIPLE CHOICE

Complete each question by circling the best answer.

1. What age group seeks orthodontic care?

   a. Adolescents
   b. Teenagers
   c. Young adults
   d. All of the above

2. What could be a genetic cause for malocclusion?

   a. A parent with a small jaw
   b. Ectopic eruption
   c. Fetal molding
   d. Thumb sucking

3. What is the term used for abnormal occlusion?

   a. Distoclusion
   b. Mesioclusion
   c. Malocclusion
   d. Facialocclusion

4. What tooth is used to determine a person's occlusion?

   a. Maxillary central incisors
   b. Mandibular first premolar
   c. Mandibular first molar
   d. Maxillary first molar

5. If a person's tooth is not properly aligned with its opposing tooth, the malalignment is referred to as:

   a. overjet.
   b. crossbite.
   c. open bite.
   d. overbite.

6. If a person occludes and you cannot see the mandibular anterior teeth, he or she is diagnosed with:

   a. overjet.
   b. crossbite.
   c. open bite.
   d. overbite.

7. What position(s) will the orthodontist evaluate for facial symmetry?

   a. Frontal view
   b. Distal view
   c. Profile view
   d. a and c

8. What type of radiograph is most commonly exposed in orthodontics?

   a. Periapical
   b. Cephalometric
   c. Panoramic
   d. Bite-wing

9. How many photographs are commonly taken in a records appointment?

   a. Two
   b. Four
   c. Five
   d. Six

10. What gypsum material is most commonly used for fabricating orthodontic diagnostic models?

    a. Plaster
    b. Stone
    c. Alginate
    d. Polyether

11. What instrument is part of the setup for seating and cementing a molar band?

    a. Howe pliers
    b. Bite stick
    c. Scaler
    d. Hemostat

12. What is the orthodontic scaler used for?

    a. Removing calculus from bands and brackets
    b. Placing separators
    c. Tying in arch wires
    d. Removing cement

13. What is another name for 110 pliers?

    a. Contouring pliers
    b. Howe pliers
    c. Weingart pliers
    d. Band-removing pliers

14. To ease in the placement of orthodontic bands, what procedure is completed to open the contact between teeth?

    a. Wearing of a positioner
    b. Placement of a ligature tie
    c. Bonding of a bracket
    d. Placement of a separator

15. When cementing bands, what can be used to prevent cement from getting into the buccal tubes or attachments?

    a. String
    b. Chap Stick
    c. Utility wax
    d. b and c

16. How are brackets adhered to a tooth?

    a. Cement
    b. Sealant
    c. Bonding agent
    d. Wax

17. Where would most auxiliary attachments be found on braces?

    a. Brackets
    b. Arch wire
    c. Bands
    d. Retainer

18. What type of arch wire is indicated for correcting malaligned teeth?

    a. Round wire
    b. Rectangular wire
    c. Braided wire
    d. Twisted wire

19. How is an arch wire sized for a patient without placing it in his or her mouth?

    a. Cephalometric radiograph
    b. Study model
    c. Used arch wire
    d. b and c

20. Besides using ligature ties, what other technique is used to hold in an arch wire?

    a. Cement
    b. Elastomeric ties
    c. Band
    d. Positioner

21. What appliance might the orthodontist use to control growth and/or tooth movement?

    a. Space maintainer
    b. Retainer
    c. Headgear
    d. All of the above

22. How can hard foods possibly harm braces?

    a. Bend a wire
    b. Loosen a bracket
    c. Pull off a band
    d. All of the above

23. How can a patient make flossing easier with braces?

    a. Using a floss threader
    b. Use of waxed floss
    c. Use of unwaxed floss
    d. Having the arch wire positioned toward the incisal or occlusal edge

24. When braces come off, does that mean treatment is over?

    a. Yes
    b. No

25. An example of a retention appliance is the:

    a. Hawley retainer.
    b. positioner.
    c. lingual retainer.
    d. all of the above

CASE STUDY

Jeramy is 14 years old and has completed the diagnostic phase for corrective orthodontics. Through discussion with his parents and orthodontist, Jeramy has agreed to have braces placed to correct crowding in the anterior area and a crossbite on his left side. He is scheduled today to have his first and second molars banded.

1. What diagnostic tools are used to evaluate Jeramy's case?
2. Discuss the importance of having Jeramy, his parents, and the orthodontist together when making the final decision about having braces.
3. What procedure is completed on Jeramy before having bands fitted and cemented?
4. What is your role in the fitting and cementation of orthodontic bands?
5. After banding, what is the next procedure to schedule Jeramy for?

61 | Communication in the Dental Office

SHORT ANSWER QUESTIONS

1. Identify patient needs.
2. Discuss oral communications, and identify the differences between verbal and nonverbal communications.
3. Describe telephone courtesy.
4. Describe and compare the handling of different types of telephone calls.
5. Describe external and internal marketing.
6. Discuss the types of stress that exist in a dental practice.
7. Discuss how the team concept can improve communication.

FILL IN THE BLANK

Select the best term from the list below and complete the following statements.

Copier
Fax machine
Letterhead
Marketing
Nonverbal communication
Salutation
Verbal communication
Word processor

1. The part of the letter that contains the greeting is the _____.

2. _____ is the type of communication in which people use words to express themselves.

3. A _____ is a computerized business machine used to type out documents.

4. A _____ is a business machine that can make duplicates from an original.

5. A business machine that can send written or typed materials over a phone line is a

   _____.

6. _____ is the type of communication in which people use body language to express themselves.

7. The _____ is the part of a letter that contains the name and address of the person sending the letter.

8. _____ is a way of advertising or recruiting people to a business.

MULTIPLE CHOICE

Complete each question by circling the best answer.

1. Body language is what type of communication?

   a. Verbal
   b. Written
   c. Nonverbal
   d. Speech

2. What percentage of spoken words is it estimated that people never hear?

   a. 50%
   b. 75%
   c. 90%
   d. 100%

3. What nonverbal behavior shows tension and uneasiness?

   a. Restrained gait
   b. Grasping the chair arms
   c. Rapid, shallow breathing
   d. All of the above

4. Select a more professional term for pulling a tooth.

   a. Luxation
   b. Take
   c. Extract
   d. Tug

5. How is a patient psychologically influenced by the attitudes of others?

   a. From acquired fears
   b. From subjective fears
   c. From objective fears
   d. All of the above

6. How are objective fears acquired?

   a. By others expressing their experiences
   b. Through fears learned from past experiences
   c. By dreaming them up
   d. By reading about them

7. What are some of the best ways to calm an irate patient?

   a. Listening
   b. Maintaining eye contact
   c. Nodding your head
   d. All of the above

8. The most important public relations tool in a dental office is the:

   a. professional letter.
   b. fax machine.
   c. telephone.
   d. newsletter.

9. At what ring should you answer the phone?

   a. First
   b. Second
   c. Third
   d. Does not matter

10. When the dental office is closed, how are messages obtained?

    a. Answering service
    b. Answering machine
    c. E-mail
    d. a and b

11. What piece of equipment allows people to send and receive written messages?

    a. Telephone
    b. Fax machine
    c. Photocopier
    d. Pager

12. What part of a letter includes the salutation?

    a. Date
    b. Inside address
    c. Opening
    d. Closing

13. Who would you correspond with besides the patient?

    a. Other dental practices
    b. Dental associations
    c. Dental insurance companies
    d. All of the above

14. Who in the dental profession would *not* be involved in the marketing of a practice?

    a. Dentist
    b. Business assistant
    c. Dental laboratory technician
    d. Dental assistant

15. How much should a practice invest in marketing?

    a. 1% to 2% of gross revenue
    b. 3% to 5% of gross revenue
    c. 5% to 8% of gross revenue
    d. 20% of gross revenue

16. Give an example of an external marketing activity.

    a. Newsletter
    b. Attending a health fair
    c. Website
    d. All of the above

17. What is the key to a successful work environment?

    a. High salaries
    b. Teamwork
    c. Good benefits
    d. Job flexibility

18. What would *not* be a stress factor for working in a dental office?

    a. Job flexibility
    b. Overbooking of patients
    c. Multiple tasks
    d. Little job advancement

WRITTEN COMMUNICATION ACTIVITY

Type a professional letter that includes the following information.

1. Dental practice heading.
2. Addressed to patients of the practice.
3. The introduction of a new dentist to the practice.
4. How this new team member will affect scheduling within the practice.
5. Any new changes in the staff due to the addition of a new dentist.

SHORT ANSWER QUESTIONS

1. Discuss the role of the office manager/business assistant in the dental office.
2. Identify types of practice records and files.
3. Identify how these filing systems are used: alphabetical, numerical, cross-reference, chronological, and subject.
4. Describe how the business assistant schedules appointments for maximum productivity.
5. Identify three types of preventive recall systems, and state the benefits of each.
6. Describe the function of computerized practice management systems and manual bookkeeping systems.
7. Discuss the management of inventory systems.

FILL IN THE BLANK

Select the best term from the list below and complete the following statements.

Active file
Buffer time
Call list
Chronological file
Cross-reference file
Daily schedule
Downtime
File guides
Filing
Inactive file
Lead time
Ledger
Outguide
Patient of record
Purchase order
Rate of use
Reorder tags
Requisition
Shelf life
Unit time
Want list
Warranty

1. The _____ is the time estimate to allow for delays in ordering or shipping of backorder materials.

2. A(n) _____ is a file of a patient who has been seen within the past 2 to 3 years.

3. A filing system that divides materials into months and possible days of the month is

   a _____.

4. Time reserved on the schedule for emergency patients is the

   _____.

5. A(n) _____ is an insert between files that shows the letters or numbers of the patient records that follow it.

6. Files of patients that are not in constant

   use are _____.

7. A(n) _____ is a file that is listed in alphabetical order by name and gives its document number.

8. A(n) _____ is a list made up of patients who can come in for an appointment on short notice.

9. _____ is the waiting period between patient procedures.

10. Printed schedules that are copied and placed throughout the office for easy

    viewing are the _____.

11. _____ is the act of classifying and arranging records to be easily retrieved when needed.

12. A(n) _____ is a type of file or statement that contains the patient's financial records.

13. A(n) _____ is like a bookmark for a filing system.

14. A written statement outlining the manufacturer's responsibility for replacing and repair of their product

    is a(n) _____.

15. A(n) _____ is a form that authorizes the purchase of supplies from the supplier.

16. A(n) _____ is a patient of the dental practice.

17. The _____ of something is the time a product may be stored before it begins to deteriorate and is no longer usable.

18. Time increments used in planning

    appointments are _____.

19. A(n) _____ is a list of supplies to be ordered and questions to be asked of the representative.

20. The _____ is how many or how much of a product is used within a given time.

21. _____ is a formal request for supplies.

22. _____ is a notation system that indicates when the supply of a certain item is low and it needs to be reordered.

MULTIPLE CHOICE

Complete each question by circling the best answer.

1. Who is responsible for overseeing the marketing activities of a dental practice?

    a. Dentist
    b. Clinical assistants
    c. Outside company
    d. Business assistants

2. How should a new employee learn about office protocol?

    a. Through the interview
    b. Office manual
    c. Attending a continuing education course
    d. From the dentist

3. What continues to replace manual work in the operating procedures of the dental office?

    a. Temporary service
    b. Typewriter
    c. Tape recorder
    d. Computer

4. Give another term for patient statement.

    a. Patient record
    b. Ledger
    c. File
    d. Document

5. How much free space should be left on each shelf of a filing cabinet?

    a. 2 inches
    b. 4 inches
    c. 6 inches
    d. 1 foot

6. What is used to mark a space from which a file has been taken?

    a. Bookmark
    b. Empty file
    c. Ledger
    d. Outguide

7. What is the easiest filing system used?

    a. Chronological
    b. Alphabetical
    c. Numerical
    d. Color-coded

8. If a patient has not been seen within the past 3 years, what would his or her status be as a patient of the dental practice?

    a. Active
    b. On recall
    c. Backorder
    d. Inactive

9. How many minutes make up one unit of time for scheduling?

    a. 5 to 7 minutes
    b. 10 to 15 minutes
    c. 20 to 30 minutes
    d. 60 minutes

10. What elements should be outlined in an appointment book?

    a. Office hours
    b. Buffer times
    c. Meetings
    d. All of the above

11. If a patient does not keep his or her appointment, where should this be recorded?

    a. Ledger
    b. Patient record
    c. Appointment book
    d. Patient statement

12. What is the most common period of time for recall appointments?

    a. 3 months
    b. 6 months
    c. 9 months
    d. 1 year

13. If a patient is seen in April, what is his or her recall time?

    a. August
    b. September
    c. October
    d. November

14. What factors must be determined when a product needs to be reordered?

    a. Rate of use
    b. Shelf life
    c. Lead time
    d. All of the above

15. How is an item marked for reorder?

    a. Reorder tag
    b. Blue slip
    c. Outguide
    d. Inguide

16. How are supplies ordered?

    a. From a sales representative
    b. On the Internet
    c. From a catalog
    d. All of the above

17. What happens when an item is not available from a supply company?

    a. Referred to another company
    b. Call other offices for the product
    c. Go on backorder
    d. Wait until a new shipment is received

18. What would *not* be considered an expendable item?

    a. Handpiece
    b. Plastic suction tip
    c. Patient napkin
    d. Gloves

BUSINESS ACTIVITY

As the business assistant in the office, your job is to organize and maintain the operating systems of the dental practice. During your weekly team meeting, the dentist has expressed a concern for the decline of patients being seen. Because of this decrease, the revenue of the practice has decreased.

1. Does this issue concern the clinical or business staff of the practice?
2. How could the decrease in revenue affect the staff?
3. Describe how the following systems could increase the number of daily patients that are now patients of the practice.
    a. scheduling
    b. recall
    c. broken appointments
    d. quality assurance
4. Describe different methods to increase the number of new patients in the practice.

63 | Financial Management of the Dental Office

SHORT ANSWER QUESTIONS

1. Describe the role of computerized practice management systems.
2. Describe how manual bookkeeping systems work.
3. Describe how financial arrangements can be set up with a patient.
4. Describe the importance of collections in the dental office.
5. Explain the policy that a business assistant should follow regarding check writing.
6. Explain the purpose of business summaries.
7. Describe payroll withholding taxes, and discuss the financial responsibility of the employer for them.
8. Describe the role that dental insurance plays in a patient's treatment.
9. Define insurance fraud.
10. List the parties involved with dental insurance.
11. Give the types of prepaid dental programs.
12. Define managed care.
13. Explain dual coverage.
14. Explain how dental procedures and coding are used in filing.
15. Describe the procedure and purpose of a claim forms follow-up.

FILL IN THE BLANK

Select the best term from the list below and complete the following statements.

Accounting
Accounts payable
Audit trail
Bonding
Bookkeeping
Carrier
CDT
Change fund

Check
Check register
Coordination of benefits (COB)
Customary
Deposit slip
Disbursements
Expenses
Fixed overhead
Gross income
Invoice
Ledger
Net income
Packing slip
Payee
Pegboard system
Petty cash
Posted
Provider
Reasonable
Responsible party
Statement
Transaction
Usual
Walkout statement

1. Expenses and disbursements paid from a business are called _____.

2. The _____ is a method of tracking the accuracy and completeness of bookkeeping records.

3. The process of managing financial accounts of a business is _____.

4. The _____ is a fixed amount of cash.

5. A(n) _____ is a draft or an order on a bank for payment of a specific amount of money.

6. _____ is the means to pay out on an account.

7. _____ is the overhead of a business to keep operating.

8. A(n) _____ is a record of all checks issued and deposits made on a specific account.

9. _____ is a system that is designed to maintain financial records of a business.

10. A dentist will have _____, which is a form of insurance that reimburses an employer for a loss resulting from theft by an employee.

11. The _____ coordinates insurance coverage between two insurance carriers.

12. A fee that is within the range of the usual fee charged for a service is the _____ fee.

13. A(n) _____ is an itemized memorandum of the money to be deposited into the bank.

14. A(n) _____ is the insurance company that pays the claims and collects premiums.

15. _____ are procedure codes that are assigned to dental services for the process of dental insurance.

16. _____ is the total money of all professional income received.

17. A(n) _____ is an itemized list of goods specifying the prices and terms of sale.

18. A financial statement that maintains all account transactions is a(n) _____.

19. _____ is income minus the expenses that are taken out.

20. The _____ is an itemized listing of shipped goods.

21. Ongoing business expenses are _____.

22. The _____ is the person's name on the check as the recipient of the amount shown.

23. _____ is a term used for documenting money transactions within a business.

24. The _____ is the dentist who provides treatment to a patient.

25. A fee that the dentist charges for a specific service is considered a _____ fee.

26. The _____ is similar to a receipt in that it gives an account balance.

27. A fee that is considered fair for an extensive or complex treatment is called _____.

28. The person who has agreed to pay for an account is considered the _____.

29. A manual bookkeeping system is the _____.

30. A small amount of cash that is kept on hand for small daily expenses is _____.

31. A(n) _____ is a summary of all charges, payments, credits, and debits for the month.

32. A(n) _____ is a change in payment or an adjustment made to a financial account.

MULTIPLE CHOICE

Complete each question by circling the best answer.

1. What type(s) of bookkeeping systems are used in a dental practice?

   a. Accounts receivable
   b. Accounts payable
   c. Accounts taxable
   d. a and b

2. What form will you use to gather financial information from a patient?

   a. Treatment plan
   b. Consent form
   c. Registration form
   d. Ledger

3. Where should the business assistant discuss financial arrangements with a patient?

   a. Dental treatment area
   b. Dental lab
   c. Reception area
   d. Private setting

4. Money that is owed to the practice is considered:

   a. accounts payable.
   b. revenue.
   c. accounts receivable.
   d. gross income.

5. If a dental office does not have a computerized accounts receivable system, what would be used?

   a. Calculator
   b. Word processor
   c. Pegboard system
   d. Ledger

6. What form is used to transmit a patient's fee from the treatment area to the business office?

   a. Receipt
   b. Patient record
   c. Ledger
   d. Charge slip

7. What common means of payment can a patient use for his or her account?

   a. Cash
   b. Credit
   c. Insurance
   d. All of the above

8. How often should bank deposits be made?

   a. Daily
   b. Weekly
   c. Monthly
   d. Quarterly

9. When should an office begin collection efforts on a past due account?

   a. 15 days
   b. 30 days
   c. 60 days
   d. 90 days

10. How can a business follow through on the collection of fees?

    a. Letters
    b. Phone call
    c. Collection agency
    d. All of the above

11. An example of fixed overhead is:

    a. dental supplies.
    b. continuing education.
    c. salaries.
    d. business supplies.

12. A paycheck is a person's:

    a. gross income.
    b. net income.
    c. reimbursement.
    d. accounts receivable.

13. What documents are received with a shipment of supplies?

    a. Packing slip
    b. Invoice
    c. Statement
    d. All of the above

14. C.O.D. means:

    a. cancel order delivered.
    b. cost of dental service.
    c. cash on delivery.
    d. cash order delinquent.

15. Where do you record checks and deposits made on an account?

    a. Daily schedule
    b. Check register
    c. Recall system
    d. Patient registration

16. What term indicates that an account does not have enough money to cover a check?

    a. Insufficient funds
    b. Bounced
    c. Inadequate funds
    d. Delinquent

17. The most commonly used method(s) of calculating fee-for-service benefits are:

    a. usual.
    b. customary.
    c. reasonable.
    d. all of the above

18. What is the specified amount of money that an insured person must pay before his or her insurance goes into effect?

    a. Overhead
    b. Deductible
    c. Customary fee
    d. Reimbursement fee

19. A child or spouse of an insurance subscriber is considered to be:

    a. uninsured.
    b. a co-payer.
    c. a dependent.
    d. deductible.

20. A patient's insurance is submitted through:

    a. a fax.
    b. registered mail.
    c. a claim form.
    d. a table of allowances.

INSURANCE ACTIVITY

On the following insurance form complete the following information.

Dental Claim Form

See reverse for instructions

1. ☐ Dentist's pre-treatment estimate ☐ Dentist's statement of actual services Provider ID #	2. ☐ Medicaid Claim ☐ EPSDT Prior Authorization # Patient ID #	3. **Carrier name and address**

PATIENT COVERAGE INFORMATION

4. Patient name first m.i. last	5. Relationship to employee ☐ self ☐ child ☐ spouse ☐ other _____	6. Sex m f	7. Patient birthdate MM DD YYYY	8. If full time student school city

9. Employee/subscriber name and mailing address	10. Employee/subscriber dental plan I.D. number	11. Employee/subscriber birthdate MM DD YYYY	12. Employer (company) name and address	13. Group number

14. Is patient covered by another dental plan yes no If yes, complete 15-a. Is patient covered by a medical plan? yes no	15-a. Name and address of carrier(s)	15-b. Group no.(s)	16. Name and address of other employer(s)

17-a. Employee/subscriber name (if different from patient's)	17-b. Employee/subscriber dental plan I.D. number	17-c. Employee/subscriber birthdate MM DD YYYY	18. Relationship to patient ☐ self ☐ parent ☐ spouse ☐ other _____

19. I have reviewed the following treatment plan and fees. I agree to be responsible for all charges for dental services and materials not paid by my dental benefit plan, unless the treating dentist or dental practice has a contractual agreement with my plan prohibiting all or a portion of such charges. To the extent permitted under applicable law, I authorize release of any information relating to this claim.

❯ _____
Signed (Patient* – see reverse)   Date

20. I hereby authorize payment of the dental benefits otherwise payable to me directly to the below named dental entity.

❯ _____
Signed (Employee/subscriber)   Date

BILLING DENTIST

21. Name of Billing Dentist or Dental Entity	30. Is treatment result of occupational illness or injury?	No	Yes	If yes, enter brief description and dates

22. Address where payment should be remitted	31. Is treatment result of auto accident?			

23. City, State, Zip	32. Other accident?			

24. Dentist Soc. Sec. or T.I.N. (see reverse**)	25. Dentist license no.	26. Dentist phone no.	33. If prosthesis, is this initial placement?	(If no, reason for replacement)	34. Date of prior placement

27. First visit date current series	28. Place of treatment Office Hosp. ECF Other	29. Radiographs or models enclosed? No Yes How many?	35. Is treatment for orthodontics?	If service already commenced enter:	Date appliances placed	Mos. treatment remaining

36. Identify missing teeth with "x"

37. Examination and treatment plan – List in order from tooth no. 1 through tooth no. 32 – Using charting system shown.

For administrative use only

Tooth # or letter	Surface	Description of service (including x-rays, prophylaxis, materials used, etc.)	Date service performed Mo. Day Year	Procedure number	Fee

38. Remarks for unusual services

39. I hereby certify that the procedures as indicated by date have been completed and that the fees submitted are the actual fees I have charged and intend to collect for those procedures.

❯ _____
Signed (Treating Dentist)   License Number   Date

40. Address where treatment was performed
                                City   State   Zip

41. Total Fee Charged	
42. Payment by other plan	
Max. Allowable	
Deductible	
Carrier %	
Carrier pays	
Patient pays	

©**American Dental Association, 1994**
J510   (Same as ADA Dental Claim Form - J504, J511, J512)

Personal information:

Birth date:	5-22-79
Soc. Sec. #:	402-38-285
Name:	Jason F. Scott
Address:	8402 Alexander Drive Colorado Springs, CO 39720
Home Phone:	486-555-1847
Employer:	US Olympic Association
Work Phone:	486-555-4910

Responsible Party:

Same as above

Dental Insurance Information:

Name of Insured:	Jason F. Scott
Insurance Company:	Dental Support
Group #:	48204
Employee Certificate #:	40238285–20
Address:	P.O. Box 313 Denver, CO
Annual Benefits:	1800.00

Treatment to be Recorded:

Date	Tooth and Surface	Treatment	Fee
3/12/01		Periodic Oral Evaluation	75.00
3/12/01		Full Mouth Series	65.00
3/12/01		Oral Prophylaxis	80.00
4/29/01	3 MOD	Amalgam	90.00
4/29/01	4 DO	Amalgam	60.00
5/03/01	10 F	Composite	32.00
5/03/01	11 DI	Composite	64.00
6/10/01	20	Root Canal	700.00
6/20/01	20	PFM Crown	800.00

64 | Marketing Your Skills

SHORT ANSWER QUESTIONS

1. Describe your career goals in the profession of dental assisting.
2. What types of potential career opportunities are available for you?
3. Describe how to prepare a job interview.
4. Discuss factors to consider in salary negotiations.
5. Discuss the elements of an employment agreement.
6. Describe the steps for achieving career objectives.
7. Describe the steps for job termination.

MULTIPLE CHOICE

Complete each question by circling the best answer.

1. What would not be an employment opportunity that a dental assistant may choose?

   a. Teaching
   b. Sales
   c. Dental hygiene
   d. Office administration

2. Where would you most commonly see a job position for a dental assistant?

   a. Newspaper
   b. Dental assisting program
   c. Dental society newsletter
   d. All of the above

3. What is the most common means of communication for your first contact with a future employer?

   a. Letter
   b. Telephone
   c. Fax
   d. E-mail

4. A cover letter:

   a. gives your educational background.
   b. describes your past work experience.
   c. covers your resume.
   d. introduces you.

5. What item(s) should not be included in a resume?

   a. Marital status
   b. Race
   c. Religion
   d. All of the above

6. How long should a resume be?

   a. Paragraph
   b. One page
   c. Two pages
   d. Does not matter

7. The most critical part of an interview is:

   a. the first time you talk on the phone.
   b. the first ten minutes.
   c. discussing the salary.
   d. the closing remarks.

8. What time frame is routinely considered provisional employment?

   a. First week
   b. First month
   c. After a few months
   d. First year

9. Termination without notice or severance pay is considered:

   a. summary dismissal.
   b. negligence.
   c. discrimination.
   d. unprofessional.

10. What is the most important factor in gaining professional success?

    a. Amount of money you make
    b. You like the people around you
    c. Having a positive attitude
    d. Your professional title

ACTIVITY

1. Prepare a cover letter to be used for seeking employment.
2. Prepare a resume to be used for seeking employment.

Competency 10-1	Identify the Major Landmarks and Structures of the Face

Performance Objective: The student will demonstrate the ability to locate and identify the following landmarks of the face by carefully pointing to these structures on another student.

Grading Criteria:

    __3__   Student meets most of the criteria without assistance

    __2__   Student requires assistance to meet the stated criteria

    __1__   Student did not prepare accordingly for the stated criteria

    __0__   Not applicable

Criteria	Peer	Self	Instructor	Comment
1. Identified the ala of the nose.				
2. Identified the inner canthus and outer canthus of the eye.				
3. Identified the commissure of the lips.				
4. Identified the location of the frontal sinuses.				
5. Identified the location of the maxillary sinuses.				
6. Identified the location of the parotid glands.				
7. Identified the philtrum.				
8. Identified the tragus of the ear.				
9. Identified the vermilion border.				
10. Identified the zygomatic arch.				

Total amount of points earned _____

Grade _____ *Instructor's initials* _____

Competency 10-2	Locate and Identify the Major Landmarks, Structures, and Normal Tissues of the Mouth

Performance Objective: The student will be able to locate and identify the following landmarks of the mouth.

Grading Criteria:

   3   Student meets most of the criteria without assistance

   2   Student requires assistance to meet the stated criteria

   1   Student did not prepare accordingly for the stated criteria

   0   Not applicable

Note: Once the student has learned appropriate infection control measures, a mouth mirror and tongue blade should be used to perform this procedure on a classmate.

Criteria	Peer	Self	Instructor	Comment
1. Located the dorsum of the tongue.				
2. Located the area of the gag reflex.				
3. Identified the hard and soft palates.				
4. Identified the gingival margin.				
5. Located the incisive papilla.				
6. Identified the mandibular labial frenum.				
7. Identified the maxillary labial frenum.				
8. Located the sublingual frenum.				
9. Identified the vestibule of the mouth.				
10. Located Wharton's duct.				

Total amount of points earned _____

Grade _____ *Instructor's initials* _____

Competency 11-1	Identify the Primary and Permanent Dentition According to the Universal and the Fédération Dentaire Internationale (FDI) Numbering Systems

Performance Objective: The student will be able to identify all of the teeth according to the Universal and FDI numbering systems.

Grading Criteria:

   __3__   Student meets most of the criteria without assistance

   __2__   Student requires assistance to meet the stated criteria

   __1__   Student did not prepare accordingly for the stated criteria

   __0__   Not applicable

Criteria	Peer	Self	Instructor	Comment
1. Identified the primary teeth in each arch according to the Universal Numbering System.				
2. Identified the primary teeth in each arch according to the FDI Numbering System.				
3. Identified the permanent teeth in each arch according to the Universal Numbering System.				
4. Identified the permanent teeth in each arch according to the FDI Numbering System.				

Total amount of points earned _____

Grade _____ *Instructor's initials* _____

Competency 12-1	Identify the Surfaces of Anterior and Posterior Teeth

Performance Objective: The student will be able to identify and name the surfaces of the anterior and posterior teeth.

Grading Criteria:

    __3__   Student meets most of the criteria without assistance

    __2__   Student requires assistance to meet the stated criteria

    __1__   Student did not prepare accordingly for the stated criteria

    __0__   Not applicable

Criteria	Peer	Self	Instructor	Comment
1. Identified the surfaces of the maxillary anterior teeth.				
2. Identified the surfaces of the maxillary posterior teeth.				
3. Identified the surfaces of the mandibular anterior teeth.				
4. Identified the surfaces of the mandibular posterior teeth.				

Total amount of points earned _____

Grade _____   *Instructor's initials* _____

Competency 15-1

Applying Topical Fluoride Gel or Foam

Performance Objective: The student will demonstrate the ability to apply a topical fluoride gel or foam.

Grading Criteria:

    3   Student meets most of the criteria without assistance

    2   Student requires assistance to meet the stated criteria

    1   Student did not prepare accordingly for the stated criteria

    0   Not applicable

Criteria	Peer	Self	Instructor	Comment
1. Selected appropriate tray and other materials.				
2. Dispensed appropriate amount of fluoride material into the tray.				
3. Positioned the patient and provided patient instructions.				
4. Dried the teeth.				
5. Inserted the tray and placed cotton rolls between the arches.				
6. Promptly placed the saliva ejector and tilted the patient's head forward.				
7. Removed the tray without allowing the patient to rinse or swallow.				
8. Used the saliva ejector or HVE tip to remove excess saliva and solution.				
9. Instructed the patient not to rinse, eat, drink, or brush the teeth for at least 30 minutes.				

Total amount of points earned _____

Grade _____   *Instructor's initials* _____

Competency
15-2

Assist the Patient With Dental Floss

Performance Objective: The student will demonstrate the ability to assist a patient in learning how to use dental floss.

Grading Criteria:

    __3__   Student meets most of the criteria without assistance

    __2__   Student requires assistance to meet the stated criteria

    __1__   Student did not prepare accordingly for the stated criteria

    __0__   Not applicable

Criteria	Peer	Self	Instructor	Comment
1. Dispensed appropriate amount of dental floss.				
2. Stretched the floss tightly between the fingers and used the thumb and index finger to guide the floss into place.				
3. Held the floss tightly between the thumb and forefinger of each hand.				
4. Passed the floss gently between the teeth.				
5. Curved the floss into a C-shape against each tooth, and wiped up and down against the tooth surfaces.				
6. Repeated these steps on each side of all the teeth in both arches.				
7. Moved a fresh piece of floss into the working position as the floss became frayed or soiled.				
8. Used a bridge threader to floss under any fixed bridges.				

Total amount of points earned _____

Grade _____ *Instructor's initials* _____

Competency 19-2	Handwashing Prior to Gloving

Performance Objective: The student will demonstrate the proper technique for handwashing before gloving.

Grading Criteria:

__3__	Student meets most of the criteria without assistance
__2__	Student requires assistance to meet the stated criteria
__1__	Student did not prepare accordingly for the stated criteria
__0__	Not applicable

Criteria	Peer	Self	Instructor	Comment
1. Removed all jewelry, including watch and rings.				
2. Used the foot or electronic control to regulate the flow of water. (If this was not available, used a paper towel to grasp the faucets to turn them on and off. Discarded the towel after use.)				
3. Used liquid soap, dispensed with a foot-activated or an electronic device.				
4. Vigorously rubbed together the lathered hands under a stream of water to remove surface debris.				
5. Dispensed additional soap and vigorously rubbed together the lathered hands for a minimum of 10 seconds under a stream of water.				
6. Rinsed the hands with cool water.				
7. Used a paper towel to thoroughly dry the hands and then the forearms.				

Total amount of points earned _____

Grade _____   *Instructor's initials* _____

| Competency 19-3 | Put on Personal Protective Equipment for Use During Patient Care |

Performance Objective: The student will demonstrate putting on appropriate personal protective equipment for use during patient care.

Grading Criteria:

__3__	Student meets most of the criteria without assistance
__2__	Student requires assistance to meet the stated criteria
__1__	Student did not prepare accordingly for the stated criteria
__0__	Not applicable

Note: See chapter to review for this competency.

Criteria	Peer	Self	Instructor	Comment
1. Put on fresh gown.				
2. Put on protective eyewear.				
3. Placed mask around neck, ready to be positioned on the face.				
4. Washed and dried hands, then put on exam gloves.				
5. Tucked cuff of sleeves into the gloves.				

Total amount of points earned _____

Grade _____   *Instructor's initials* _____

Competency 20-1

Place and Remove Surface Barriers

Performance Objective: The student will demonstrate the placement and removal of surface barriers.

Grading Criteria:

3	Student meets most of the criteria without assistance
2	Student requires assistance to meet the stated criteria
1	Student did not prepare accordingly for the stated criteria
0	Not applicable

Criteria	Peer	Self	Instructor	Comment
Placement of Surface Barriers				
1. Washed and dried hands.				
2. Assembled the appropriate setup.				
3. Selected the appropriate surface barriers.				
4. Placed each barrier over the entire surface to be protected.				
Removal of Surface Barriers				
1. Wore utility gloves to remove contaminated surface barriers.				
2. Very carefully removed each cover.				
3. Discarded the used covers into the regular waste trash.				
4. Washed, disinfected, and removed utility gloves.				
5. Washed and dried hands.				

Total amount of points earned _____

Grade _____ *Instructor's initials* _____

Competency 20-2	Performing Treatment Room Cleaning and Disinfection

Performance Objective: The student will demonstrate the ability to preclean and disinfect a dental treatment room and equipment surfaces.

Grading Criteria:

   3   Student meets most of the criteria without assistance

   2   Student requires assistance to meet the stated criteria

   1   Student did not prepare accordingly for the stated criteria

   0   Not applicable

Criteria	Peer	Self	Instructor	Comment
1. Assembled the appropriate setup.				
2. Wore the appropriate personal protective eyewear.				
3. Checked to see that the precleaning-disinfecting product had been prepared correctly and was fresh. Read and followed the manufacturer's instructions.				
4. Sprayed the paper towel or gauze pad with the product and vigorously wiped the surface.				
5. Sprayed a fresh paper towel or gauze pad with the product.				
6. Allowed the surface to remain moist for the manufacturer's recommended time.				

Total amount of points earned _____

Grade _____ *Instructor's initials* _____

Competency 20-3 | Disinfect an Alginate Impression

Performance Objective: The student will demonstrate the ability to disinfect an alginate impression.

Grading Criteria:

    3   Student meets most of the criteria without assistance

    2   Student requires assistance to meet the stated criteria

    1   Student did not prepare accordingly for the stated criteria

    0   Not applicable

Note: Disinfecting applies to many aspects of dental care.

Criteria	Peer	Self	Instructor	Comment
1. Assembled the appropriate setup.				
2. Wore the appropriate personal protective eyewear.				
3. Gently cleaned the impression.				
4. Rinsed the impression and removed excess water.				
5. Sprayed the impression thoroughly with the disinfectant.				
6. Wrapped the impression loosely in a plastic bag for the recommended contact time.				
7. After the sufficient contact time, rinsed the impression.				

Total amount of points earned _____

Grade _____ Instructor's initials _____

Competency 21-1

Operating the Ultrasonic Cleaner

Performance Objective: When provided with appropriate materials, the student will demonstrate the ability to preclean instruments prior to sterilization using the ultrasonic cleaner.

Grading Criteria:

    3   Student meets most of the criteria without assistance

    2   Student requires assistance to meet the stated criteria

    1   Student did not prepare accordingly for the stated criteria

    0   Not applicable

Criteria	Peer	Self	Instructor	Comment
1. Wore appropriate personal protective eyewear.				
2. Removed the lid from the container and checked the level of solution.				
3. Placed instruments or cassette into the basket.				
4. Replaced the lid and turned the cycle to "ON."				
5. After cleaning cycle, removed the basket and rinsed the instruments.				
6. Emptied the basket onto the towel.				
7. Replaced the lid on the ultrasonic cleaner.				

Total amount of points earned _____

Grade _____   *Instructor's initials* _____

Competency 21-3

Prepare and Autoclave Instruments

Performance Objective: When provided with the appropriate materials, the student will demonstrate the ability to prepare and autoclave instruments.

Grading Criteria:

__3__ Student meets most of the criteria without assistance

__2__ Student requires assistance to meet the stated criteria

__1__ Student did not prepare accordingly for the stated criteria

__0__ Not applicable

Criteria	Peer	Self	Instructor	Comment
1. Wore appropriate personal protective eyewear.				
2. Dried instruments.				
3. Dipped nonstainless instruments and burs in a corrosion inhibitor.				
4. Placed the process indicator into the package.				
5. Packaged, sealed, and labeled the instruments.				
6. Placed, bagged, and sealed items in the autoclave.				
7. Tilted glass or metal canisters at an angle.				
8. Placed larger packs at the bottom of the chamber.				
9. Did not overload the autoclave.				
10. Followed the manufacturer's instructions.				
11. Checked the level of the water. (If necessary, added additional distilled water.)				
12. Set the autoclave controls for the appropriate time, temperature, and pressure.				

Competency 21-3 continued

Criteria	Peer	Self	Instructor	Comment
13. At the end of the sterilization cycle, vented the steam into the room, and allowed the contents of the autoclave to dry and cool.				
14. Checked the external process indicator for color change.				
15. Removed the instruments when they were cool and dry.				

Total amount of points earned _____

Grade _____   *Instructor's initials* _____

| Competency 21-4 | Prepare and Sterilize Instruments by Chemical Vapor |

Performance Objective: Given appropriate materials, the student will demonstrate the ability to prepare and sterilize instruments by chemical vapor.

Grading Criteria:

__3__	Student meets most of the criteria without assistance
__2__	Student requires assistance to meet the stated criteria
__1__	Student did not prepare accordingly for the stated criteria
__0__	Not applicable

Criteria	Peer	Self	Instructor	Comment
1. Wore appropriate personal protective eyewear.				
2. Dried the instruments.				
3. Wrapped the instruments.				
4. Packages were not too large.				
5. Read and followed the manufacturer's instructions.				
6. Read the information on the MSDS sheet for the chemical liquid.				
7. Loaded the sterilizer.				
8. Set the controls for the proper time and temperature.				
9. Followed the manufacturer's instructions for venting and cooling.				
10. Checked the external process indicator for color change.				
11. Removed the instruments when they were cool and dry.				

Total amount of points earned _____

Grade _____   *Instructor's initials* _____

Competency 21-5	Prepare and Sterilize Instruments by Dry Heat

Performance Objective: Given the appropriate materials, the student will demonstrate the ability to prepare and sterilize instruments by dry heat.

Grading Criteria:

   3   Student meets most of the criteria without assistance

   2   Student requires assistance to meet the stated criteria

   1   Student did not prepare accordingly for the stated criteria

   0   Not applicable

Criteria	Peer	Self	Instructor	Comment
1. Wore appropriate personal protective eyewear.				
2. Dried the instruments before wrapping.				
3. Opened hinged instruments.				
4. Wrapped instruments.				
5. Read and followed the manufacturer's instructions.				
6. Loaded the instruments into the dry heat chamber.				
7. Set the time and temperature.				
8. Did not place additional instruments in the load once the sterilization cycle had begun.				
9. Allowed the packs to cool before handling.				
10. Checked the indicators for color change.				

Total amount of points earned _____

Grade _____ *Instructor's initials* _____

Competency 23-1	Create an Appropriate Label for a Secondary Container

Performance Objective: The student will demonstrate using information from a Material Safety Data Sheet (MSDS) to complete a chemical label for a secondary container.

Grading Criteria:

   3   Student meets most of the criteria without assistance

   2   Student requires assistance to meet the stated criteria

   1   Student did not prepare accordingly for the stated criteria

   0   Not applicable

Criteria	Peer	Self	Instructor	Comment
1. Wrote the manufacturer's name and address on the label.				
2. Wrote the name of the chemical(s) on the label.				
3. Wrote the appropriate health hazard code in the blue triangle.				
4. Wrote the appropriate flammability and explosion hazard code in the red triangle.				
5. Wrote the appropriate reactivity code in the yellow triangle.				
6. Wrote the appropriate specific hazard warning in the white triangle.				

Total amount of points earned _____

Grade _____ *Instructor's initials* _____

Competency 26-1, 26-2	Registering a New Patient and Obtaining a Medical and Dental History

Performance Objective: The student will use the appropriate forms to gather patient registration and medical history information.

Grading Criteria:

    _3_   Student meets most of the criteria without assistance

    _2_   Student requires assistance to meet the stated criteria

    _1_   Student did not prepare accordingly for the stated criteria

    _0_   Not applicable

Criteria	Peer	Self	Instructor	Comment
1. Explained to the patient the need for this information and asked the patient to complete the forms.				
2. Provided the patient with a pen and the forms on a clipboard. Asked if the patient would like help in completing the forms.				
3. If the patient answered yes, offered to aid him or her in completing the form.				
4. Reviewed the completed forms to determine if there were questions that were not answered.				
5. Lightly circled answers to questions that required clarification.				
6. In a private setting, such as the treatment room, asked the patient about information that was not clear.				
7. If indicated, placed a medical alert label or signal inside the patient's record.				

Total amount of points earned _____

Grade _____ *Instructor's initials* _____

		Competency	
		27-1 through 27-5	Obtain and Record Vital Signs

Performance Objective: The student will obtain and record the patient's vital signs.

Grading Criteria:

	3	Student meets most of the criteria without assistance
	2	Student requires assistance to meet the stated criteria
	1	Student did not prepare accordingly for the stated criteria
	0	Not applicable

Criteria	Peer	Self	Instructor	Comment
1. **Appearance.** Observed and noted the patient's appearance, speech, and gait as he or she entered the treatment room.				
2. **Setup.** Had the correct equipment set up for the procedure.				
3. **Pulse.** Let the patient sit quietly for a few minutes, then took and recorded patient's pulse correctly.				
4. **Respiration.** Took and recorded the patient's respiration rate correctly.				
5. **Temperature.** Took and recorded the patient's oral temperature correctly.				
6. **Blood pressure.** Took and recorded the patient's blood pressure correctly.				
7. Maintained patient comfort throughout.				

Total amount of points earned _____

Grade _____   *Instructor's initials* _____

Competency 28-2

Charting of Teeth

Performance Objective: When provided with a patient chart and colored pencils, the student will demonstrate the ability to record the dentist's findings as dictated during an examination.

Grading Criteria:

3	Student meets most of the criteria without assistance
2	Student requires assistance to meet the stated criteria
1	Student did not prepare accordingly for the stated criteria
0	Not applicable

Criteria	Peer	Self	Instructor	Comment
1. Assembled the appropriate setup.				
2. Accurately recorded findings as dictated by the dentist using the symbols and abbreviations preferred by the dentist.				
3. During the periodontal probing, recorded the findings as dictated by the dentist.				
4. Accurately read back the dentist's findings.				

Total amount of points earned _____

Grade _____   *Instructor's initials* _____

| Competency 28-4 | Recording of the Completed Dental Treatment |

Performance Objective: The student will record dental treatment and services accurately, completely, and legibly.

Grading Criteria:

   __3__ Student meets most of the criteria without assistance

   __2__ Student requires assistance to meet the stated criteria

   __1__ Student did not prepare accordingly for the stated criteria

   __0__ Not applicable

Criteria	Peer	Self	Instructor	Comment
1. Made all entries in black ink.				
2. Entries were legible.				
3. Entries were made in the proper sequence.				
4. Tooth numbers were correct.				
5. Tooth surfaces were correct.				
6. All treatment entries were recorded accurately.				
7. Was able to read back entries accurately.				

Total amount of points earned _____

Grade _____ *Instructor's initials* _____

Competency 31-5	Maintain Emergency Drugs in the Dental Office

Performance Objective: Provided with a suitable emergency kit, the student will identify and state the use and route of administration for each of the drugs.

Grading Criteria:

__3__ Student meets most of the criteria without assistance

__2__ Student requires assistance to meet the stated criteria

__1__ Student did not prepare accordingly for the stated criteria

__0__ Not applicable

Note: See chapter to review for this competency.

Criteria	Peer	Self	Instructor	Comment
1. Located the emergency kit(s).				
2. Located the **epinephrine** in the drug kit, stated its use and route of administration.				
3. Located the **antihistamine** in the drug kit, stated its use and route of administration.				
4. Located the **anticonvulsant** in the drug kit, stated its use and route of administration.				
5. Located the **analgesic** in the drug kit, stated its use and route of administration.				
6. Located the **vasopressor** in the drug kit, stated its use and route of administration.				
7. Located the **antihypoglycemic** in the drug kit, stated its use and route of administration.				
8. Located the **nitroglycerin** in the drug kit, stated its use and route of administration.				
9. Located the **bronchodilator** in the drug kit, stated its use and route of administration.				
10. Located the **ammonia inhalant** in the drug kit, stated its use and route of administration.				

Total amount of points earned _____

Grade _____ *Instructor's initials* _____

| Competency 31-6 | Manage Medical Emergencies With a Conscious Patient |

Performance Objective: The student will respond appropriately to patients experiencing hyperventilation, an asthmatic attack, a localized allergic reaction, an angina attack, a potential acute myocardial infarction, and hyperglycemia.

Grading Criteria:

__3__	Student meets most of the criteria without assistance
__2__	Student requires assistance to meet the stated criteria
__1__	Student did not prepare accordingly for the stated criteria
__0__	Not applicable

Note: See chapter tables to review for this competency.

Criteria	Peer	Self	Instructor	Comment
1. Identified **hyperventilation** by the signs and symptoms, and described the care of the patient.				
2. Identified an **asthmatic attack** by the signs and symptoms, and described the care of the patient.				
3. Identified a **localized allergic reaction** by the signs and symptoms, and described the care of the patient.				
4. Identified **angina pectoris** by the signs and symptoms, and described the care of the patient.				
5. Identified a **potential acute myocardial infarction** by the signs and symptoms, and described the care of the patient.				
6. Identified **hyperglycemia** by the signs and symptoms, and described the care of the patient.				

Total amount of points earned _____

Grade _____ *Instructor's initials* _____

Competency 31-7	Manage Medical Emergencies With a Partially Conscious Patient

Performance Objective: The student will respond appropriately to patients experiencing a partial airway obstruction or a petit mal seizure.

Grading Criteria:

   3   Student meets most of the criteria without assistance

   2   Student requires assistance to meet the stated criteria

   1   Student did not prepare accordingly for the stated criteria

   0   Not applicable

Note: See chapter tables to review for this competency.

Criteria	Peer	Self	Instructor	Comment
1. Identified a partial airway obstruction by the signs and symptoms, and described the care of the patient.				
2. Identified a petit mal seizure by the signs and symptoms, and described the care of the patient.				

Total amount of points earned _____

Grade _____ *Instructor's initials* _____

Competency 31-8	Manage Medical Emergencies With an Unconscious Patient

Performance Objective: The student will respond appropriately to patients experiencing syncope, postural hypotension, anaphylaxis, hypoglycemia, a possible cerebrovascular accident, and a grand mal seizure.

Grading Criteria:

    3   Student meets most of the criteria without assistance

    2   Student requires assistance to meet the stated criteria

    1   Student did not prepare accordingly for the stated criteria

    0   Not applicable

Note: See chapter tables to review for this competency.

Criteria	Peer	Self	Instructor	Comment
1. Identified **syncope** by the signs and symptoms, and described the care of the patient.				
2. Identified **hypotension** by the signs and symptoms, and described the care of the patient.				
3. Identified **anaphylaxis** by the signs and symptoms, and described the care of the patient.				
4. Identified **hypoglycemia** by the signs and symptoms, and described the care of the patient.				
5. Identified a **potential cerebrovascular accident** by the signs and symptoms, and described the care of the patient.				
6. Identified a **grand mal seizure** by the signs and symptoms, and described the care of the patient.				

Total amount of points earned _____

Grade _____ *Instructor's initials* _____

Competency
33-2

Seating the Patient

Performance Objective: The student will determine that the treatment room is ready and will then seat and prepare the patient for treatment.

Grading Criteria:

    __3__ Student meets most of the criteria without assistance

    __2__ Student requires assistance to meet the stated criteria

    __1__ Student did not prepare accordingly for the stated criteria

    __0__ Not applicable

Criteria	Peer	Self	Instructor	Comment
1. Treatment room was properly cleaned and prepared, with the chair properly positioned and the patient's path clear.				
2. Placed instrument setup and materials in the treatment room and determined that the patient's records, radiographs, and laboratory work were in place.				
3. Identified and greeted the patient accordingly.				
4. Escorted the patient to the treatment room.				
5. Placed the patient's personal items in a safe place near the treatment room.				
6. Properly seated the patient.				
7. Placed the patient's napkin around the patient's neck.				
8. Properly positioned the dental chair for the procedure.				
9. Adjusted the operating light and then turned it on.				
10. Maintained patient comfort throughout these preparations.				

Total amount of points earned _____

Grade _____   *Instructor's initials* _____

Competency 33-7 | Assist During an Oral Examination

Performance Objective: The student will demonstrate the ability to assist during an oral examination.

Grading Criteria:

__3__ Student meets most of the criteria without assistance

__2__ Student requires assistance to meet the stated criteria

__1__ Student did not prepare accordingly for the stated criteria

__0__ Not applicable

Note: See chapter to review for this competency.

Criteria	Peer	Self	Instructor	Comment
1. Assembled the appropriate setup.				
2. Observed the patient as he or she entered the treatment room and made notations of any variations from normal.				
3. Seated, draped, and positioned patient.				
4. Anticipated the dentist's needs by transferring the correct instruments and materials.				
5. Adjusted the light as necessary.				
6. Accurately recorded findings as dictated by the dentist.				
7. At the conclusion of the procedure, dismissed the patient.				
8. Maintained patient comfort and followed appropriate infection control measures throughout the procedure.				

Total amount of points earned _____

Grade _____ *Instructor's initials* _____

Competency
33-8

Perform Single-Handed and Specialized Instrument Transfers and Exchanges

Performance Objective: The student will perform single-handed and specialized instrument transfer in a safe and efficient manner.

Grading Criteria:

   3   Student meets most of the criteria without assistance

   2   Student requires assistance to meet the stated criteria

   1   Student did not prepare accordingly for the stated criteria

   0   Not applicable

Criteria	Peer	Self	Instructor	Comment
Single-Handed Transfer and Exchange				
1. Retrieved the instrument from the instrument tray opposite the working end.				
2. Held the instrument in the transfer zone, 8 to 10 inches away from the dentist.				
3. Anticipated the dentist's transfer signal and positioned the new instrument parallel to the instrument in the dentist's hand.				
4. Retrieved the used instrument using the last two fingers.				
5. Delivered the new instrument to the dentist.				
6. Maintained safety throughout the transfer.				
Nonlocking Cotton Pliers Transfer				
1. Held the contents (cotton pellet) securely by pinching the beaks together.				
2. Delivered the pliers so the dentist could hold the beaks together.				
3. Retrieved the pliers without dropping the cotton pellet.				

Competency 33-8 continued

Criteria	Peer	Self	Instructor	Comment
Forceps Transfer				
1. Used the right hand to pick up the forceps and hold it for delivery in the position of use.				
2. Used the left hand to take the used instrument from the dentist.				
3. Delivered the new instrument to the dentist in the appropriate position.				
4. Returned the used instrument to its proper position on the tray.				
Handpiece Exchange				
1. Used the left hand to pick up the handpiece and hold it for delivery in the position of use.				
2. Used the right hand to take the used instrument from the dentist.				
3. Delivered the handpiece to the dentist in the appropriate position.				
4. When exchanging two handpieces, did not tangle the cords.				
Air-Water Syringe Transfer				
1. Held the nozzle of the air-water syringe in the delivery fingers.				
2. Retrieved the instrument the dentist was using, then delivered the syringe.				
Scissors Transfer				
1. Picked up the scissors and held them near the working end with the beaks slightly open.				
2. Positioned handles of the scissors over the dentist's fingers.				
3. Received used scissors with the beaks in the closed position.				

Total amount of points earned _____

Grade _____   *Instructor's initials* _____

Competency 33-9

Dismiss a Patient After Treatment

Performance Objective: The student will dismiss the patient after treatment.

Grading Criteria:

    __3__   Student meets most of the criteria without assistance

    __2__   Student requires assistance to meet the stated criteria

    __1__   Student did not prepare accordingly for the stated criteria

    __0__   Not applicable

Note: See chapter to review for this competency.

Criteria	Peer	Self	Instructor	Comment
1. Alerted the patient and then slowly returned the chair to an upright and low position.				
2. Provided post-treatment instructions as necessary.				
3. Removed the patient's napkin.				
4. Removed gloves and washed hands.				
5. Returned personal belongings to the seated patient.				
6. Raised the chair arm and, if necessary, assisted the patient from the chair.				
7. Directed or escorted the patient to the business office.				
8. Maintained patient comfort throughout these steps.				

Total amount of points earned _____

Grade _____   *Instructor's initials* _____

| Competency 34-1 through 34-4 | Prepare a Tray Setup for a Dental Procedure |

Performance Objective: Given a procedure, the student will gather the appropriate instruments and supplies.

Grading Criteria:

   3   Student meets most of the criteria without assistance

   2   Student requires assistance to meet the stated criteria

   1   Student did not prepare accordingly for the stated criteria

   0   Not applicable

Note: The student is provided with an appropriate assortment of instruments and supplies to choose from.

Criteria	Peer	Self	Instructor	Comment
1. Reviewed the patient record and determined the type of procedure to set up for.				
2. Described the materials and additional supplies to be set out.				
3. Gathered the instruments and placed them in the appropriate order on the tray.				
4. Prepared the materials and supplies to be readied for procedure.				
5. Stated which items required sterilization before use.				

Total amount of points earned _____

Grade _____ *Instructor's initials* _____

Competency 35-1, 35-2 | Identification and Attachment of Handpieces and Rotary Instruments

Performance Objective: Given instructions for which size and/or type to select, the student will place and remove burs in a high-speed and a low-speed handpiece.

Grading Criteria:

    3   Student meets most of the criteria without assistance

    2   Student requires assistance to meet the stated criteria

    1   Student did not prepare accordingly for the stated criteria

    0   Not applicable

Note: The student is provided with an appropriate assortment of burs and handpieces to work with.

Criteria	Peer	Self	Instructor	Comment
1. Selected the specified size and type of bur for the high-speed handpiece.				
2. Placed the bur in the handpiece in accordance with the manufacturer's instructions.				
3. Removed the bur from the handpiece in accordance with the manufacturer's instructions.				
4. Selected the specified size and type of bur for the low-speed handpiece.				
5. Placed the bur in the handpiece in accordance with the manufacturer's instructions.				
6. Removed the bur from the handpiece in accordance with the manufacturer's instructions.				

Total amount of points earned _____

Grade _____ *Instructor's initials* _____

Competency 36-1	Positioning the HVE During a Procedure

Performance Objective: The student will maintain moisture control, access, and visibility during patient care by appropriately positioning the HVE.

Grading Criteria:

   _3_   Student meets most of the criteria without assistance

   _2_   Student requires assistance to meet the stated criteria

   _1_   Student did not prepare accordingly for the stated criteria

   _0_   Not applicable

Criteria	Peer	Self	Instructor	Comment
1. Assumed correct seated position to accommodate the left- or right-handed dentist.				
2. HVE correctly positioned for the maxillary left posterior treatment.				
3. HVE correctly positioned for the maxillary right posterior quadrant.				
4. HVE correctly positioned for the mandibular left posterior treatment.				
5. HVE correctly positioned for the mandibular right posterior treatment.				
6. HVE correctly positioned for the anterior treatment with lingual access.				
7. HVE correctly positioned for the anterior treatment with facial access.				
8. Maintained patient comfort and followed appropriate infection control measures throughout.				

Total amount of points earned _____

Grade _____   *Instructor's initials* _____

Competency 36–2

Performing a Mouth Rinse

Performance Objective: The student will perform a limited-area rinse and a complete mouth rinse using the high-volume oral evacuator (HVE) and air-water syringe.

Grading Criteria:

__3__	Student meets most of the criteria without assistance
__2__	Student requires assistance to meet the stated criteria
__1__	Student did not prepare accordingly for the stated criteria
__0__	Not applicable

Criteria	Peer	Self	Instructor	Comment
Limited-Area Rinse				
1. Held the air-water syringe in the left hand.				
2. Held the HVE in the right hand using a proper grasp.				
3. Positioned the HVE in the area being worked on, and rinsed and suctioned the area.				
4. Maintained patient comfort and followed appropriate infection control measures throughout.				
Complete Mouth Rinse				
1. Held the air-water syringe in the left hand.				
2. Held the HVE in the right hand using a proper grasp.				
3. Positioned the HVE in the vestibule of mouth and, starting at one area, rinsed the mouth thoroughly, suctioning the accumulated water and debris.				
4. Maintained patient comfort and followed appropriate infection control measures throughout.				

Total amount of points earned _____

Grade _____   *Instructor's initials* _____

Competency 36-3

Place and Remove Cotton Rolls

Performance Objective: The student will place, and properly remove, cotton roll isolation for each area of the mouth.

Grading Criteria:

   3   Student meets most of the criteria without assistance

   2   Student requires assistance to meet the stated criteria

   1   Student did not prepare accordingly for the stated criteria

   0   Not applicable

Criteria	Peer	Self	Instructor	Comment
1. Placed and removed cotton rolls for the maxillary anterior isolation.				
2. Placed and removed cotton rolls for the maxillary posterior isolation.				
3. Placed and removed cotton rolls and auxiliary aids for mandibular anterior isolation.				
4. Placed and removed cotton rolls and auxiliary aids for mandibular posterior isolation.				
5. Maintained patient comfort and followed appropriate infection control measures throughout.				

Total amount of points earned _____

Grade _____ *Instructor's initials* _____

Competency
36-4

Preparing the Dental Dam

Performance Objective: The student will place and stabilize the dental dam.

Grading Criteria:

__3__	Student meets most of the criteria without assistance
__2__	Student requires assistance to meet the stated criteria
__1__	Student did not prepare accordingly for the stated criteria
__0__	Not applicable

Criteria	Peer	Self	Instructor	Comment
1. Prepared appropriate setup.				
2. Punched the dam for the teeth to be isolated.				
3. Selected the clamp and tied a ligature to it.				
4. Placed prepared clamp in dental dam forceps in the position of use.				
5. Seated clamp so that it is secure around the anchor tooth.				
6. Slid the dam down over the clamp, making sure to pull the ligature through the keyhole of the dam.				
7. Positioned the dental dam frame correctly, making sure to fastened all notches to the dam.				
8. Slid dam through all contacts using floss to push dam interproximally.				
9. Inverted the dental dam using floss, air, or a blunted instrument.				
10. Dam was ligated and stabilized.				

Competency 36-4 continued

Criteria	Peer	Self	Instructor	Comment
11. Maintained patient comfort and followed appropriate infection control measures throughout the procedure.				

Total amount of points earned _____

Grade _____   *Instructor's initials* _____

Competency 36-5

Removing the Dental Dam

Performance Objective: The student will remove the dental dam.

Grading Criteria:

    __3__   Student meets most of the criteria without assistance

    __2__   Student requires assistance to meet the stated criteria

    __1__   Student did not prepare accordingly for the stated criteria

    __0__   Not applicable

Criteria	Peer	Self	Instructor	Comment
1. Removed stabilization ligature and saliva ejector.				
2. Cut dental dam septum with scissors.				
3. Removed dental dam clamp, dental dam frame, and the used dental dam.				
4. Checked used dental dam for tears or missing pieces.				
5. Used the air-water syringe and HVE tip to rinse the patient's mouth.				
6. Used tissue to gently wipe debris from area around the patient's mouth.				
7. Maintained patient comfort and followed appropriate infection control measures throughout the procedure.				

Total amount of points earned _____

Grade _____   *Instructor's initials* _____

Competency 37-1	Applying a Topical Anesthetic

Performance Objective: The student will select the necessary setup, identify the injection site, and apply topical anesthetic.

Grading Criteria:

   3   Student meets most of the criteria without assistance

   2   Student requires assistance to meet the stated criteria

   1   Student did not prepare accordingly for the stated criteria

   0   Not applicable

Criteria	Peer	Self	Instructor	Comment
Preparation				
1. Gathered the appropriate setup.				
2. Used a sterile cotton-tipped applicator to remove a small amount of topical anesthetic ointment from the container, then replaced the cover immediately.				
3. Explained the procedure to the patient.				
4. Determined the injection site.				
5. Wiped the injection site dry using a sterile 2 × 2 gauze sponge.				
Placement				
1. Applied topical anesthetic ointment to the injection site only.				
2. Left the topical anesthetic ointment in contact with the oral tissues for 2 to 5 minutes only.				
3. Removed the cotton-tipped applicator just before the injection by the dentist.				

Competency 37-1 continued

Criteria	Peer	Self	Instructor	Comment
4. Maintained patient comfort and followed appropriate infection control measures throughout the procedure.				

Total amount of points earned _____

Grade _____   *Instructor's initials* _____

Competency 37-2	Assembling the Local Anesthetic Syringe

Performance Objective: The student will select the necessary setup and prepare an aspirating-type syringe for local anesthetic injection.

Grading Criteria:

__3__	Student meets most of the criteria without assistance
__2__	Student requires assistance to meet the stated criteria
__1__	Student did not prepare accordingly for the stated criteria
__0__	Not applicable

Criteria	Peer	Self	Instructor	Comment
Preliminary Steps				
1. Gathered the necessary setup, washed hands, and put on fresh exam gloves.				
2. Inspected the syringe, needle, and anesthetic cartridge and then prepared the syringe out of the patient's sight.				
3. Double-checked the anesthetic cartridge to confirm the anesthetic is the type the dentist ordered.				
Attach the Needle				
1. Removed the plastic cap from the syringe end of the needle, and screwed the needle onto the syringe.				
2. Loosened the colored plastic cap from the injection end of the needle.				
Insert the Cartridge				
1. Retracted the piston using the thumb ring, then inserted the anesthetic cartridge with the rubber stopper end first.				
2. Released the piston and gently engaged the harpoon.				
3. Gently pulled back on the thumb ring to be certain the harpoon was securely in place.				

Competency 37-2 continued

Criteria	Peer	Self	Instructor	Comment
Transfer the Syringe				
1. Transferred the syringe below the patient's chin or behind the patient's head as instructed.				
2. Took appropriate safety precaution measures while transferring the syringe.				
Disassemble the Used Syringe				
1. Retracted the piston of the syringe by pulling back on the thumb ring.				
2. While still retracting the piston, removed the anesthetic cartridge from the syringe.				
3. Unscrewed and removed the needle from the syringe.				
4. Disposed of the needle in an appropriate sharps container.				
5. Disposed of the used cartridge in the appropriate manner.				
6. Followed appropriate infection control measures throughout the procedure.				

Total amount of points earned _____

Grade _____   *Instructor's initials* _____

| Competency 37-4 | Assisting in the Administration and Monitoring of Nitrous Oxide (N_2O) Sedation |

Performance Objective: The student will assist the dentist with the administration of nitrous oxide analgesia by monitoring the patient's reactions and recording appropriate information in the patient's record.

Grading Criteria:

    3   Student meets most of the criteria without assistance

    2   Student requires assistance to meet the stated criteria

    1   Student did not prepare accordingly for the stated criteria

    0   Not applicable

Criteria	Peer	Self	Instructor	Comment
Before Administration				
1. Checked the nitrous oxide and oxygen tanks for adequate supply.				
2. Gathered appropriate supplies and placed a sterile mask of the appropriate size on the tubing.				
3. Updated the patient's health history, then took and recorded the patient's blood pressure and pulse.				
4. Familiarized the patient with the experience of nitrous oxide analgesia.				
5. Placed the patient in a supine position.				
6. Assisted the patient with placement of the mask.				
7. Made necessary adjustments to the mask and tubing to ensure proper fit.				
During Administration				
1. At the dentist's direction, adjusted the flow of oxygen to the established tidal volume.				
2. At the dentist's direction, adjusted the flow of nitrous oxide and oxygen.				

Competency 37-4 continued

Criteria	Peer	Self	Instructor	Comment
3. Noted on the patient's chart the time and volumes of gas needed to achieve baseline.				
4. Monitored the patient throughout the procedure.				
Oxygenation				
1. At the dentist's direction, turned off the flow of nitrous oxide and increased the flow of oxygen.				
2. After oxygenation was complete, removed the nosepiece, then slowly returned the patient to the upright position.				
3. After the patient was dismissed, recorded on the patient's record the concentrations of gases administered and any unusual patient reactions to the analgesia.				
4. Maintained patient comfort and followed appropriate infection control measures.				

Total amount of points earned _____

Grade _____   *Instructor's initials* _____

<table>
<tr><td></td><td>Manual Processing of Dental Radiographs</td></tr>
</table>

| Competency 39-2 | Manual Processing of Dental Radiographs |

Performance Objective: The student will demonstrate the ability to process films manually.

Grading Criteria:

__3__	Student meets most of the criteria without assistance
__2__	Student requires assistance to meet the stated criteria
__1__	Student did not prepare accordingly for the stated criteria
__0__	Not applicable

Criteria	Peer	Self	Instructor	Comment
Preparation Steps				
1. Followed all of the infection control steps.				
2. Stirred the solutions, checked solution levels and their temperature. The temperature was between 65° and 70°F.				
3. Labeled the film rack with the patient's name and the date of exposure.				
4. Washed and dried hands and put on gloves.				
5. Turned on the safelight, then turned off the white light.				
6. Opened the film packets and allowed the films to drop onto the clean paper towel. Used care not to touch the films.				
7. Removed contaminated gloves and washed and dried hands.				
Processing Steps				
1. Attached each film to the film rack so that films were parallel and not touching each other.				
2. Agitated the rack slightly while inserting it into the solution.				
3. Started the timer. The timer was set according to the manufacturer's instructions on the basis of the temperature of the solutions.				

Competency 39-2 continued

Criteria	Peer	Self	Instructor	Comment
4. Removed the rack of films, after the timer went off, and rinsed it in the running water in the center tank for 20 to 30 seconds.				
5. Determined the fixation time and set the timer. Immersed the rack of films in the fixer tank.				
6. Returned the rack of films to the center tank with circulating water for a minimum of 20 minutes.				
7. Removed the rack of films from the water and allowed it to dry.				
8. When completely dry, removed the films from the rack and mounted them in an appropriately labeled mount.				

Total amount of points earned _____

Grade _____   *Instructor's initials* _____

Competency 39-3	Processing Films in an Automatic Film Processor

Performance Objective: The student will be able to process films using an automatic processor.

Grading Criteria:

    3   Student meets most of the criteria without assistance

    2   Student requires assistance to meet the stated criteria

    1   Student did not prepare accordingly for the stated criteria

    0   Not applicable

Criteria	Peer	Self	Instructor	Comment
1. Turned on the machine and allowed the chemicals to warm up, according to the manufacturer's recommendations for proper temperature before the machine was operational.				
2. Followed the infection control steps.				
3. Removed the black paper and lead foil. Placed the films into the processor.				
4. Fed the films slowly into the machine and kept them straight. Allowed at least 10 seconds between inserting each film into the processor before inserting the next film. Alternated slots within the processor when possible.				

Total amount of points earned _____

Grade _____ *Instructor's initials* _____

Competency 40-1 | Practicing Infection Control During Film Exposure

Performance Objective: The student will demonstrate the ability to implement appropriate infection control protocol during film exposure.

Grading Criteria:
　　　　　__3__ Student meets most of the criteria without assistance
　　　　　__2__ Student requires assistance to meet the stated criteria
　　　　　__1__ Student did not prepare accordingly for the stated criteria
　　　　　__0__ Not applicable

Criteria	Peer	Self	Instructor	Comment
1. Washed and dried hands, and placed barriers.				
2. Washed and dried hands, and put on gloves.				
3. Wiped the exposed packet on the paper towel.				
4. When finished exposing films and while still gloved, discarded the paper towel.				
5. Removed gloves and washed hands before leaving the treatment room.				
6. Carried the *cup* or *bag* of exposed films to the processing area.				

Total amount of points earned _____

Grade _____   *Instructor's initials* _____

Competency 40-2

Infection Control When in the Darkroom

Performance Objective: The student will be able to implement proper infection control in the darkroom.

Grading Criteria:

      3   Student meets most of the criteria without assistance

      2   Student requires assistance to meet the stated criteria

      1   Student did not prepare accordingly for the stated criteria

      0   Not applicable

Criteria	Peer	Self	Instructor	Comment
1. Placed a paper towel and a clean cup on the counter near the processor.				
2. Put on a new pair of gloves.				
3. Opened the film packets and allowed each exposed film to drop onto the paper towel. Unwrapped films did not come into contact with the gloves.				
4. Removed the lead foil from the packet and placed it into the foil container.				
5. Placed the empty film packets into the clean cup.				
6. Discarded the cup, and removed gloves with inside turned out and discarded them.				
7. Placed the films into the processor or on developing racks with bare hands.				

Total amount of points earned _____

Grade _____ *Instructor's initials* _____

| Competency | Practicing Infection Control When |
| 40-3 | Using the Daylight Loader |

Performance Objective: The student will be able to practice infection control techniques while using the daylight loader.

Grading Criteria:

__3__	Student meets most of the criteria without assistance
__2__	Student requires assistance to meet the stated criteria
__1__	Student did not prepare accordingly for the stated criteria
__0__	Not applicable

Criteria	Peer	Self	Instructor	Comment
1. Washed and dried hands, then placed a paper towel or piece of plastic as a barrier inside the bottom of the daylight loader.				
2. Placed the cup with the contaminated film, a clean pair of gloves, and a second paper cup on the barrier, and closed the top.				
3. Put clean hands through the sleeves and put on the gloves.				
4. Opened the packets and allowed the films to drop onto the clean barrier, placed the contaminated packets into the second cup, and the lead foil into the foil container.				
5. After opening the last packet, removed gloves with insides turned out, and inserted the films into the developing slots.				
6. After inserting the last film, pulled ungloved hands through sleeves.				

Competency 40-3 continued

Criteria	Peer	Self	Instructor	Comment
7. Opened the top of the loader, and carefully pulled the ends of the barrier over the paper cup and used gloves and discarded. Used care not to touch the contaminated parts of the barrier with bare hands.				
8. Washed and dried hands.				

Total amount of points earned _____

Grade _____   *Instructor's initials* _____

Competency
41-2

Assembling the XCP (Extension–Cone
Paralleling) Instruments

Performance Objective: The student will demonstrate the ability to assemble a localizer ring type of film-holding instrument.

Grading Criteria:
     3   Student meets most of the criteria without assistance
     2   Student requires assistance to meet the stated criteria
     1   Student did not prepare accordingly for the stated criteria
     0   Not applicable

Criteria	Peer	Self	Instructor	Comment
1. Assembled the instruments for the area to be radiographed.				
2. Placed the film into the backing plate.				
3. Used the entire horizontal length of the bite-block.				
4. Placed the anterior edge of the bite-block on the incisal or occlusal surfaces of the teeth being radiographed.				
5. Instructed the patient to close slowly but firmly.				
6. Placed a cotton roll between the bite-block and the teeth of the opposite arch.				
7. Moved the localizer ring down the indicator rod into position.				
8. Aligned the position-indicator device.				
9. Exposed the film, then removed the film and holding device from the patient's mouth.				

Total amount of points earned _____

Grade _____ *Instructor's initials* _____

Competency 41-3	Exposure of a Full-Mouth Survey Using the Paralleling Technique

Performance Objective: The student will be able to produce a full-mouth radiographic survey using the paralleling technique.

Grading Criteria:

      _3_   Student meets most of the criteria without assistance

      _2_   Student requires assistance to meet the stated criteria

      _1_   Student did not prepare accordingly for the stated criteria

      _0_   Not applicable

Criteria	Peer	Self	Instructor	Comment
Preparation				
1. Determined the number and type of films to be exposed.				
2. Labeled a paper cup or plastic bag, and placed it outside of the room where the x-ray machine is used.				
3. Turned on the x-ray machine and checked the basic settings.				
4. Washed hands.				
5. Dispensed the desired number of films and stored them outside of the room where the x-ray machine is used.				
6. Placed all necessary barriers.				
Positioning the Patient				
1. Seated the patient in the dental chair.				
2. Positioned the patient's head.				
3. Asked the patient to remove eyeglasses and bulky earrings.				
4. Draped the patient with a lead apron and thyroid collar.				
5. Washed hands and put on clean exam gloves.				
6. Asked the patient to remove any removable prosthetic appliances from his or her mouth.				

Competency 41-3 continued

Criteria	Peer	Self	Instructor	Comment
7. Opened the package and assembled the sterile film-holding instruments.				
8. Used a mouth mirror to inspect the oral cavity.				

Maxillary Central/Lateral Incisor Region

1. Inserted the film packet vertically into the anterior block.				
2. Positioned the film.				
3. Instructed the patient to close slowly but firmly.				
4. Positioned the localizing ring and position-indicator device (PID), and then exposed the film.				

Maxillary Cuspid Region

1. Inserted the film packet vertically into the anterior bite-block.				
2. Positioned the film packet with the cuspid and first premolar centered.				
3. Instructed the patient to close slowly but firmly.				
4. Positioned the localizing ring and PID, and then exposed the film.				

Maxillary Premolar Region

1. Inserted the film packet horizontally into the posterior bite-block.				
2. Centered the film packet on the second premolar.				
3. With the instrument and film in place, instructed the patient to close slowly but firmly.				
4. Positioned the localizing ring and PID, and then exposed the film.				

Competency 41-3 *continued*

Criteria	Peer	Self	Instructor	Comment
Maxillary Molar Region				
1. Inserted the film packet horizontally into the posterior bite-block.				
2. Centered the film packet on the second molar.				
3. With the instrument and film in place, instructed the patient to close slowly but firmly.				
4. Positioned the localizing ring and PID, then exposed the radiograph.				
Mandibular Incisor Region				
1. Inserted the film packet vertically into the anterior bite-block.				
2. Centered the film packet between the central incisors.				
3. With the instrument and film in place, instructed the patient to close slowly but firmly.				
4. Positioned the localizing ring and PID, then exposed the film.				
Mandibular Cuspid Region				
1. Inserted film packet vertically into the anterior bite-block.				
2. Centered the film on the cuspid.				
3. Used a cotton roll between the maxillary teeth and bite-block, if necessary.				
4. With the instrument and film in place, instructed the patient to close slowly but firmly.				
5. Positioned the localizing ring and PID, then exposed the film.				
Mandibular Premolar Region				
1. Inserted the film horizontally into the posterior bite-block.				

Competency 41-3 continued

Criteria	Peer	Self	Instructor	Comment
2. Centered the film on the contact point between the second premolar and first molar.				
3. With the instrument and film in place, instructed the patient to close slowly but firmly.				
4. Positioned the localizing ring and PID, then exposed the film.				
Mandibular Molar Region				
1. Inserted the film horizontally into the posterior bite-block.				
2. Centered the film on the second molar.				
3. With the instrument and film in place, instructed the patient to close slowly but firmly.				
4. Positioned the localizing ring and PID, then exposed the film.				

Total amount of points earned _____

Grade _____   *Instructor's initials* _____

Competency
41-5

Producing a Four-Film Bite-Wing
Survey

Performance Objective: The student will be able to produce a four-film bite-wing survey.

Grading Criteria:

      __3__ Student meets most of the criteria without assistance

      __2__ Student requires assistance to meet the stated criteria

      __1__ Student did not prepare accordingly for the stated criteria

      __0__ Not applicable

Criteria	Peer	Self	Instructor	Comment
1. Placed the film in the patient's mouth for a premolar film.				
2. Positioned the film in proper position.				
3. Set the vertical angulation.				
4. Positioned horizontal angulation.				
5. Positioned the position indicator device.				

Total amount of points earned _____

Grade _____ *Instructor's initials* _____

Competency 41-6	Producing Maxillary and Mandibular Occlusal Radiographs

Performance Objective: The student will demonstrate the ability to produce a maxillary and mandibular occlusal radiograph on either a patient or a mannequin.

Grading Criteria:

    __3__ Student meets most of the criteria without assistance

    __2__ Student requires assistance to meet the stated criteria

    __1__ Student did not prepare accordingly for the stated criteria

    __0__ Not applicable

Criteria	Peer	Self	Instructor	Comment
Maxillary Occlusal Technique				
1. Positioned the patient's head so the film plane was parallel to the floor.				
2. Placed the film packet in the patient's mouth with the white side of the film on the occlusal surfaces of the maxillary teeth.				
3. Placed the film as far posterior as possible.				
4. Positioned the position-indicator device (PID) so that the central ray was directed at a 65-degree angle through the bridge of the nose to the center of the film packet.				
5. Pressed the x-ray machine-activating button and made the exposure.				
Mandibular Occlusal Technique				
1. Tilted the patient's head back to a comfortable position. The midsagittal plane was vertical.				
2. Placed the film packet in the patient's mouth with the white side of the film on the occlusal surfaces of the mandibular teeth.				
3. Positioned the film as far posterior as possible.				

Competency 41-6 continued

Criteria	Peer	Self	Instructor	Comment
4. Positioned the PID so that the central ray was directed at 90 degrees (right angle) to the center of the film packet.				
5. Pressed the x-ray machine-activating button and made the exposure.				

Total amount of points earned _____

Grade _____   *Instructor's initials* _____

Competency	
41-7	*Mounting Dental Radiographs*

Performance Objective: The student will be able to mount a full-mouth series of radiographs.

Grading Criteria:

   __3__   Student meets most of the criteria without assistance

   __2__   Student requires assistance to meet the stated criteria

   __1__   Student did not prepare accordingly for the stated criteria

   __0__   Not applicable

Criteria	Peer	Self	Instructor	Comment
1. Hands were clean and dry before radiographs were handled. Films were grasped only at the edges, never on the front or back.				
2. Selected the appropriate-size mount, and labeled it with the patient's name and the date that the radiographs were exposed.				
3. Arranged the dried radiographs in anatomic order on a piece of clean white paper or on a flat view box.				
4. Once the films were arranged properly, placed them neatly in the mount.				

Total amount of points earned _____

Grade _____ *Instructor's initials* _____

Competency 43-3	Mixing Intermediate Restorative Material

Performance Objective: The student will assemble the necessary supplies, then correctly manipulate the material for placement into a Class I cavity preparation.

Grading Criteria:

   _3_   Student meets most of the criteria without assistance

   _2_   Student requires assistance to meet the stated criteria

   _1_   Student did not prepare accordingly for the stated criteria

   _0_   Not applicable

Note: In states where it is legal, the assistant may place the temporary restoration in a prepared tooth.

Criteria	Peer	Self	Instructor	Comment
1. Selected the proper material and assembled the appropriate supplies.				
2. Dispensed materials in the proper sequence and quantities, then immediately recapped the containers.				
3. Incorporated the powder and liquid according to the manufacturer's directions.				
4. Completed the mix within the appropriate working time.				
5. Completed mix was appropriate consistency for a temporary restoration.				
6. When finished, cared for supplies and materials appropriately.				

Total amount of points earned _____

Grade _____   *Instructor's initials* _____

Competency
44-1

Apply Calcium Hydroxide to Prepared Tooth Surface

Performance Objective: The student will assemble the necessary supplies, then correctly manipulate the material for use as a cavity liner.

Grading Criteria:

   __3__ Student meets most of the criteria without assistance

   __2__ Student requires assistance to meet the stated criteria

   __1__ Student did not prepare accordingly for the stated criteria

   __0__ Not applicable

Note: In states where it is legal, the assistant may place the cavity liner in a prepared tooth.

Criteria	Peer	Self	Instructor	Comment
1. Selected the proper material and assembled the appropriate supplies.				
2. Dispensed materials in the proper sequence and quantities, then immediately recapped the containers.				
3. Incorporated the pastes according to the manufacturer's directions.				
4. Completed the mix within the appropriate working time.				
5. Wiped instrument clean, then transferred the applicator to the operator holding the paper pad with the mix in the transfer zone.				
6. When finished, cared for supplies and materials appropriately.				

Total amount of points earned _____

Grade _____ *Instructor's initials* _____

Competency
44-9

Mix Zinc Oxide Eugenol for a Base

Performance Objective: The student will assemble the necessary supplies, then correctly manipulate the material for use as a base.

Grading Criteria:

__3__	Student meets most of the criteria without assistance
__2__	Student requires assistance to meet the stated criteria
__1__	Student did not prepare accordingly for the stated criteria
__0__	Not applicable

Note: See chapter to review for this competency.

Criteria	Peer	Self	Instructor	Comment
As a Base				
1. Selected the proper material and assembled the appropriate supplies.				
2. Dispensed materials in the proper sequence and quantities, then immediately recapped the containers.				
3. Incorporated the powder and liquid according to the manufacturer's directions.				
4. Completed the mix within the appropriate working time.				
5. Completed mix was appropriate consistency for use as a base.				
6. When finished, cared for supplies and materials appropriately.				

Total amount of points earned _____

Grade _____ *Instructor's initials* _____

Competency 45-1	Mix Zinc Oxide Eugenol for Cementation

Performance Objective: The student will assemble the necessary supplies, then correctly manipulate mixes of the material for use in permanent cementation.

Grading Criteria:

    __3__ Student meets most of the criteria without assistance

    __2__ Student requires assistance to meet the stated criteria

    __1__ Student did not prepare accordingly for the stated criteria

    __0__ Not applicable

Criteria	Peer	Self	Instructor	Comment
For Permanent Cementation				
1. Selected the proper material and assembled the appropriate supplies.				
2. Dispensed materials in the proper sequence and quantities, then immediately recapped the containers.				
3. Incorporated the powder and liquid according to the manufacturer's directions.				
4. Completed the mix within the appropriate working time.				
5. Completed mix was appropriate consistency for permanent cementation.				
6. When finished, cared for supplies and materials appropriately.				

Total amount of points earned _____

Grade _____ *Instructor's initials* _____

Competency 45-3	Mix Zinc Phosphate for Cementation

Performance Objective: The student will assemble the necessary supplies, and then correctly manipulate the material for use in the cementation of a cast crown. The student will also be asked to place the cement inside the crown.

Grading Criteria:

    __3__ Student meets most of the criteria without assistance

    __2__ Student requires assistance to meet the stated criteria

    __1__ Student did not prepare accordingly for the stated criteria

    __0__ Not applicable

Note: If a crown is available, the student will also be asked to place the cement inside the crown.

Criteria	Peer	Self	Instructor	Comment
For Cementation				
1. Selected the proper material and assembled the appropriate supplies.				
2. Dispensed materials in the proper sequence and quantities, then immediately recapped the containers.				
3. Incorporated the powder and liquid according to the manufacturer's directions.				
4. Completed the mix within the appropriate working time.				
5. Completed mix was appropriate consistency for cementation.				
6. *Optional:* Lined crown with cement.				
7. When finished, cared for supplies and materials appropriately.				

Total amount of points earned _____

Grade _____ *Instructor's initials* _____

| Competency 45-4 | Mix Polycarboxylate Cement for Permanent Cementation |

Performance Objective: The student will assemble the necessary supplies, and then correctly manipulate the material for use in cementation.

Grading Criteria:

   _3_   Student meets most of the criteria without assistance

   _2_   Student requires assistance to meet the stated criteria

   _1_   Student did not prepare accordingly for the stated criteria

   _0_   Not applicable

Criteria	Peer	Self	Instructor	Comment
For Cementation				
1. Selected the proper material and assembled the appropriate supplies.				
2. Dispensed materials in the proper sequence and quantities, then immediately recapped the containers.				
3. Incorporated the powder and liquid according to the manufacturer's directions.				
4. Completed the mix within the appropriate working time.				
5. Completed mix was appropriate consistency for cementation				
6. When finished, cared for supplies and materials appropriately.				

Total amount of points earned _____

Grade _____ *Instructor's initials* _____

Competency 45-5	Mix Glass Jonomer for Permanent Cementation

Performance Objective: The student will assemble the necessary supplies, and then correctly manipulate the material for use in the cementation of a cast crown.

Grading Criteria:

   3   Student meets most of the criteria without assistance

   2   Student requires assistance to meet the stated criteria

   1   Student did not prepare accordingly for the stated criteria

   0   Not applicable

Note: If a crown is available, the student will also be asked to place the cement inside the crown.

Criteria	Peer	Self	Instructor	Comment
1. Selected the proper material and assembled the appropriate supplies.				
2. Dispensed materials in the proper sequence and quantities, then immediately recapped the containers.				
3. Incorporated the powder and liquid according to the manufacturer's directions.				
4. Completed the mix within the appropriate working time.				
5. Completed mix was appropriate consistency for cementation.				
6. *Optional:* Lined crown with cement.				
7. When finished, cared for supplies and materials appropriately.				

Total amount of points earned _____

Grade _____ *Instructor's initials* _____

Competency 45-7	Cement Removal from a Permanent and Temporary Cementation

Performance Objective: In states where it is legal, the student will remove excess cement from the coronal surfaces of a cast restoration.

Grading Criteria:

    <u> 3 </u> Student meets most of the criteria without assistance

    <u> 2 </u> Student requires assistance to meet the stated criteria

    <u> 1 </u> Student did not prepare accordingly for the stated criteria

    <u> 0 </u> Not applicable

Criteria	Peer	Self	Instructor	Comment
1. Assembled appropriate setup.				
2. Determined that the cement had set and then removed the cotton rolls.				
3. Established a firm fulcrum for the hand holding the instrument.				
4. Placed the tip of the instrument at the gingival edge of the cement and used overlapping vertical strokes (away from the gingiva) to remove the bulk of the cement.				
5. Applied slight lateral pressure (toward the tooth surface) to remove the remaining cement.				
6. Passed a length of dental floss, with knots tied in it, through the mesial and distal contact areas.				
7. Used overlapping strokes with an explorer to examine all tooth surfaces.				
8. Completed the procedure without scratching the cast restoration.				
9. Removed any remaining cement particles and then performed a complete mouth rinse.				

Competency 45-7 continued

Criteria	Peer	Self	Instructor	Comment
10. Maintained patient comfort and followed appropriate infection control measures throughout the procedure.				

Total amount of points earned _____

Grade _____   Instructor's initials _____

Competency 46-2, 46-3	Taking a Mandibular or a Maxillary Impression

Performance Objective: The student will take an alginate impression of diagnostic quality.

Grading Criteria:

    __3__ Student meets most of the criteria without assistance

    __2__ Student requires assistance to meet the stated criteria

    __1__ Student did not prepare accordingly for the stated criteria

    __0__ Not applicable

Criteria	Peer	Self	Instructor	Comment
1. Gathered appropriate supplies and seated the patient.				
2. Selected and prepared the impression tray.				
3. Used air-water syringe and HVE to rinse patient's mouth.				
4. Mixed the alginate correctly.				
5. Loaded the maxillary and mandibular tray correctly.				
6. Seated tray, completed impression, and removed tray.				
7. The completed impression showed that the tray was centered in the patient's mouth.				
8. Evaluated the impression and determined that it was acceptable.				
9. Maintained patient comfort and followed appropriate infection control measures throughout the procedure.				

Total amount of points earned _____

Grade _____ *Instructor's initials* _____

Competency 46-6

Taking a Wax-Bite Registration

Performance Objective: The student will take a wax-bite registration.

Grading Criteria:

__3__	Student meets most of the criteria without assistance
__2__	Student requires assistance to meet the stated criteria
__1__	Student did not prepare accordingly for the stated criteria
__0__	Not applicable

Note: Mandibular and maxillary impressions have already been taken on this patient.

Criteria	Peer	Self	Instructor	Comment
1. Gathered appropriate supplies.				
2. Provided patient instruction.				
3. Prepared material appropriately.				
4. Placed softened wax on occlusal surfaces of the mandibular teeth.				
5. Completed the wax-bite registration and removed it.				
6. Determined that the wax-bite registration was acceptable.				
7. Maintained patient comfort and followed appropriate infection control measures throughout the procedure.				

Total amount of points earned _____

Grade _____ *Instructor's initials* _____

Competency
46-9

Assist With a Final Impression

Performance Objective: The student will demonstrate assisting the operator in obtaining a final impression using a paste system.

Grading Criteria:

     3   Student meets most of the criteria without assistance

     2   Student requires assistance to meet the stated criteria

     1   Student did not prepare accordingly for the stated criteria

     0   Not applicable

Note: See chapter to review for this competency.

Criteria	Peer	Self	Instructor	Comment
Preparation				
1. Gathered the appropriate supplies.				
2. Determined that the tray was ready and had been painted with an adhesive.				
Preparation of Light-Bodied Material				
1. Dispensed approximately 1¼ to 2 inches of the light-bodied material onto a clean paper pad, or prepared light-bodied cartridges in the extruder gun.				
2. Incorporated the catalyst into the base paste, producing a streak-free mix.				
3. Loaded syringe with paste or from the extruder gun and completed assembly in less than 30 seconds.				
4. Passed the prepared syringe to the dentist.				
Preparation of Heavy-Bodied Material				
1. With a paste system, used a clean mixing pad and clean spatula.				

Competency 46-9 continued

Criteria	Peer	Self	Instructor	Comment
2. Extruded the tray-type base material to the appropriate length, or attached the heavy-bodied cartridges onto the extruder gun, with new extruder tips.				
3. Completed a homogeneous mix within the time recommended by the manufacturer. (This is usually 45 seconds to 1 minute.)				
4. Loaded the material into the tray correctly.				
5. Received the used syringe from the operator and passed the prepared tray.				

Total amount of points earned _____

Grade _____   *Instructor's initials* _____

Competency 48-2a	Assisting in a Class Two Amalgam Restoration

Performance Objective: In a simulated situation, the student will assist with the preparation, placement, and finishing of a class II amalgam restoration.

Grading Criteria: __3__ Student meets most of the criteria without assistance
 __2__ Student requires assistance to meet the stated criteria
 __1__ Student did not prepare accordingly for the stated criteria
 __0__ Not applicable

Criteria	Peer	Self	Instructor	Comment
1. Had setup correctly sequenced and set up.				
2. Had dental materials placed and readied.				
3. Assisted during administration of the local anesthetic solution and placement of the dental dam.				
4. Transferred instruments according to four-handed technique.				
5. Maintained visibility for the operator and used the HVE correctly.				
6. Mixed and transfer base/liner materials.				
7. Assisted with preparation and placement of the matrix band, retainer, and wedge.				
8. Mixed and transferred or expressed amalgam.				
9. Transferred carving instruments.				
10. Assisted with removal of the wedge, retainer, matrix band, and dental dam removal.				
11. Assisted during final carving and occlusal adjustment.				
12. Gave postoperative instructions to the patient.				

Competency 48-2a continued

Criteria	Peer	Self	Instructor	Comment
13. Maintained patient comfort and followed appropriate infection control measures throughout the procedure.				

Total amount of points earned _____

Grade _____   *Instructor's initials* _____

| Competency 48-2b | Assisting in a Class Two Composite Restoration |

Performance Objective: In a simulated situation, the student will assist with the preparation, placement, and finishing of a class II composite restoration.

Grading Criteria:
    __3__ Student meets most of the criteria without assistance
    __2__ Student requires assistance to meet the stated criteria
    __1__ Student did not prepare accordingly for the stated criteria
    __0__ Not applicable

Criteria	Peer	Self	Instructor	Comment
1. Prepared in sequence correct setup for procedure.				
2. Had dental materials prepared for use.				
3. Transferred instruments according to four-handed technique.				
4. Maintained visibility for the operator.				
5. Used the HVE and air-water syringe correctly.				
6. Assisted with matrix and wedge placement.				
7. Mixed and transferred base/liner materials.				
8. Assisted in the application and rinsing of etchant and bonding.				
9. Transferred or expressed composite syringe.				
10. Followed manufacturer's instructions on all materials.				
11. Maintained patient comfort and followed appropriate infection control measures throughout the procedure.				

Total amount of points earned _____

Grade _____   *Instructor's initials* _____

Competency 48-3	Assisting in a Class Three Composite Restoration

Performance Objective: In a simulated situation, the student will assist with the preparation, placement, and finishing of a class III composite restoration.

Grading Criteria:

3	Student meets most of the criteria without assistance
2	Student requires assistance to meet the stated criteria
1	Student did not prepare accordingly for the stated criteria
0	Not applicable

Criteria	Peer	Self	Instructor	Comment
1. Instruments assembled correctly and in sequence of use.				
2. Dental materials prepared and ready for use.				
3. Transferred instruments according to four-handed technique.				
4. Maintained visibility for the operator.				
5. Used the HVE and air-water syringe correctly.				
6. Assisted with matrix and wedge placement.				
7. Transferred and passed base/liner materials.				
8. Assisted in the application and rinsing of etchant and bonding.				
9. Transferred or expressed composite syringe.				
10. Followed manufacturer's instructions on all materials.				
11. Maintained patient comfort and followed appropriate infection control measures throughout the procedure.				

Total amount of points earned _____

Grade _____   *Instructor's initials* _____

Competency 49-1	Assembling the Matrix Band and Universal Retainer

Performance Objective: The student will assemble a Tofflemire retainer and band for each quadrant of the dental arch.

Grading Criteria:

    __3__ Student meets most of the criteria without assistance

    __2__ Student requires assistance to meet the stated criteria

    __1__ Student did not prepare accordingly for the stated criteria

    __0__ Not applicable

Criteria	Peer	Self	Instructor	Comment
1. Gathered the appropriate supplies.				
2. Stated which guide slot would be used for each quadrant.				
3. Determined which tooth to be treated and selected the appropriate band. Placed the middle of the band on the paper pad and burnished the band with a ball burnisher.				
4. Held the retainer so that the diagonal slot was visible and turned the outer knob clockwise until the end of the spindle was visible in the diagonal slot in the vise.				
5. Turned the inner knob counterclockwise until the vise moved next to the guide slots and the retainer was ready to receive the matrix band.				
6. Identified the occlusal and gingival aspects of the matrix band, and brought the ends of the band together to form a loop.				
7. Placed the occlusal edge of the band into the retainer first and then guided the band between the correct guide slots.				

Competency 49-1 continued

Criteria	Peer	Self	Instructor	Comment
8. Locked the band in the vise.				
9. Used the handle end of the mouth mirror to open and round the loop of the band.				
10. Adjusted the size of the loop to fit the selected tooth.				

Total amount of points earned _____

Grade _____   *Instructor's initials* _____

Competency 49-2	Placement and Removal of a Matrix Band and Wedge for a Class Two Procedure

Performance Objective: The student will place a Tofflemire retainer, matrix band, and wedge on a typodont that has a tooth with a class II amalgam preparation. The student will then remove the matrix band and retainer and wedge.

Grading Criteria:

__3__	Student meets most of the criteria without assistance
__2__	Student requires assistance to meet the stated criteria
__1__	Student did not prepare accordingly for the stated criteria
__0__	Not applicable

Criteria	Peer	Self	Instructor	Comment
Band Placement				
1. Verified correct assembly of matrix and retainer.				
2. Held the retainer parallel to the buccal surfaces of the teeth with the diagonal slot facing toward the gingiva.				
3. Placed a cotton roll between the matrix band and finger.				
4. Adjusted loop snugly around the tooth.				
5. Used an explorer to check the adaptation of the band to determine that it was firm and extended no more than 1 to 1.5 mm beyond the gingival margin of the cavity preparation.				
6. Checked to make sure that the matrix band did not extend more than 2 mm above the highest cusp of the tooth.				
7. Burnished contact with a ball burnisher.				
8. Maintained patient comfort and followed appropriate infection control measures throughout the procedure.				

Competency 49-2 continued

Criteria	Peer	Self	Instructor	Comment
Wedge Placement				
1. Selected correct size wedge.				
2. Used cotton pliers to insert the wedge from lingual embrasure so that the flat side of the wedge was toward the gingiva.				
3. Verified proximal contact and sealed gingival margin.				
4. Maintained patient comfort and followed appropriate infection control measures throughout the procedure.				
Removal Steps				
1. Placed a cotton roll between the occlusal edge of the matrix band and the index finger of one hand. With the other hand, slowly turned the outer knob of the retainer in a counterclockwise direction.				
2. Carefully slid the retainer toward the occlusal surface.				
3. Used cotton pliers to gently spread open the ends of the matrix band and gently lift the matrix band in an occlusal direction using a seesaw motion.				
4. Removed the wedge using No. 110 pliers or cotton pliers.				
5. Discarded the used matrix band in the sharps container.				
6. Maintained patient comfort and followed appropriate infection control measures throughout the procedure.				

Total amount of points earned _____

Grade _____   *Instructor's initials* _____

Competency 50–1	Placement and Removal of Gingival Retraction Cord

Performance Objective: The student will demonstrate placement, packing, and removal of gingival retraction cord.

Grading Criteria:

   _3_   Student meets most of the criteria without assistance

   _2_   Student requires assistance to meet the stated criteria

   _1_   Student did not prepare accordingly for the stated criteria

   _0_   Not applicable

Criteria	Peer	Self	Instructor	Comment
Preparation				
1. Gathered the appropriate setup.				
2. Rinsed and gently dried the prepared tooth, and isolated the quadrant with cotton rolls.				
3. Cut a piece of retraction cord 1 to 1½ inches in length, depending on the size and type of tooth under preparation.				
4. Formed a loose loop of the cord and placed the cord in the cotton pliers.				
Placement				
1. Slipped the loop of the retraction cord over the tooth so that the overlapping ends were on the facial surface of the tooth.				
2. Laid the cord into the sulcus, then used the packing instrument and working in a clockwise direction packed the cord gently but firmly into the sulcus.				
3. Used a gentle rocking movement of the instrument as the instrument moved forward to the next loose section of retraction cord. Repeated this action until the length of cord was packed in place.				

Competency 50-1 continued

Criteria	Peer	Self	Instructor	Comment
4. Overlapped the working end of the cord where it met the first end of the cord. Tucked the ends into the sulcus on the facial aspect.				
5. Left the cord in place for 5 to 7 minutes maximum. During this time, advised the patient to remain still, and kept the area dry.				

Removal

1. Grasped the end of the retraction cord with cotton pliers and removed the cord in a counterclockwise direction.				
2. If so instructed by the operator, gently dried the area and placed fresh cotton rolls.				

Total amount of points earned _____

Grade _____ *Instructor's initials* _____

Competency 50-2	Assist in a Crown and Bridge Preparation

Performance Objective: The student will assist the dentist during the preparation visit for a crown and bridge restoration.

Grading Criteria:

__3__	Student meets most of the criteria without assistance
__2__	Student requires assistance to meet the stated criteria
__1__	Student did not prepare accordingly for the stated criteria
__0__	Not applicable

Criteria	Peer	Self	Instructor	Comment
1. Prepared the appropriate setup and materials.				
2. Prepared the syringe and assisted during administration of the local anesthetic solution.				
3. Throughout the preparation, maintained a clear, well-lighted operating field.				
4. Anticipated the dentist's needs. Transferred instruments and changed burs as necessary.				
5. Stated when the final impression would be taken.				
6. Stated when provisional coverage would be placed. (In states where it is legal, after this topic has been studied the student prepares and places the provisional coverage.)				
7. Prepared the case to be sent to the laboratory.				

Competency 50-2 continued

Criteria	Peer	Self	Instructor	Comment
8. Maintained patient comfort and followed appropriate infection control measures throughout the procedure.				

Total amount of points earned _____

Grade _____   *Instructor's initials* _____

Competency 50-4 | Assist During Cementation of a Crown or Bridge Restoration

Performance Objective: The student will assist the dentist during the cementation visit of a crown or bridge restoration.

Grading Criteria:

__3__ Student meets most of the criteria without assistance

__2__ Student requires assistance to meet the stated criteria

__1__ Student did not prepare accordingly for the stated criteria

__0__ Not applicable

Note: See chapter to review for this competency.

Criteria	Peer	Self	Instructor	Comment
1. Determined in advance that the case had been returned from the laboratory.				
2. Prepared the appropriate setup and materials.				
3. Prepared the syringe and assisted during administration of the local anesthetic solution.				
4. Assisted during removal of provisional coverage. (In states where it is legal, the student removes the provisional coverage.)				
5. Anticipated the dentist's needs while the casting is tried in and adjusted.				
6. Assisted with or placed cotton rolls to isolate the quadrant and to keep the area dry.				
7. Assisted during placement of the cavity varnish or a desensitizer.				
8. At a signal from the dentist, mixed the cement, lined the internal surface of the casting with a thin coating of cement, and transferred the prepared crown to the dentist.				

Competency 50-4 *continued*

Criteria	Peer	Self	Instructor	Comment
9. Provided home care instructions to the patient.				
10. Maintained patient comfort and followed appropriate infection control measures throughout the procedure.				

Total amount of points earned _____

Grade _____   *Instructor's initials* _____

Competency
51-1

Fabrication and Cementation of a
Custom Acrylic Provisional Crown

Performance Objective: The student will prepare and place temporary coverage for a tooth prepared to receive a crown.

Grading Criteria:

    __3__ Student meets most of the criteria without assistance

    __2__ Student requires assistance to meet the stated criteria

    __1__ Student did not prepare accordingly for the stated criteria

    __0__ Not applicable

Criteria	Peer	Self	Instructor	Comment
Preliminary Impression				
1. Gathered the appropriate setup.				
2. Obtained the preliminary impression.				
Create the Provisional Coverage				
1. Isolated and dried the prepared tooth.				
2. Dispensed equal portions of base and catalyst and mixed together according to the manufacturer's directions.				
3. Placed the material in the impression in the area of the prepared tooth. Returned the impression to the mouth and allowed it to set for 2 to 2½ minutes or longer.				
4. Removed the impression from the patient's mouth, and then removed the provisional coverage from the impression.				
5. Used acrylic burs to trim the temporary coverage.				
6. Cured the provisional coverage according to the manufacturer's instructions.				

Competency 51-1 continued

Criteria	Peer	Self	Instructor	Comment
7. After curing, removed any excess material with finishing diamonds, discs, or finishing burs.				
8. Checked the occlusion and makes any adjustments using laboratory burs and disks on the provisional outside of the mouth.				
9. Completed final polishing using rubber discs and polishing lathe and pumice.				
Cementation				
1. Mixed the temporary cement and filled the crown.				
2. Seated the provisional coverage and allows the cement to set.				
3. Removed any excess cement and checked the occlusion.				
4. Had dentist check.				
5. Provided the patient with home care instructions.				
6. Maintained patient comfort and followed appropriate infection control measures throughout the procedure.				

Total amount of points earned _____

Grade _____ *Instructor's initials* _____

Competency 51-4	Fitting and Cementation of a Polycarbonate Crown

Performance Objective: The student will prepare and temporarily cement a preformed polycarbonate crown to protect a tooth that has been prepared for a full crown.

Grading Criteria:

3	Student meets most of the criteria without assistance
2	Student requires assistance to meet the stated criteria
1	Student did not prepare accordingly for the stated criteria
0	Not applicable

Criteria	Peer	Self	Instructor	Comment
Preparation				
1. Gathered the appropriate setup.				
2. Selected the appropriate shape and size crown and checked for width, length, and adaptation at the margins.				
3. Used crown and bridge scissors to reduce the height of the crown by trimming the cervical margin.				
4. Smoothed rough edges with an acrylic trimming stone or acrylic bur.				
5. Polished the edges with a Burlew wheel, or on a lathe with pumice.				
Cementation				
1. Mixed the temporary cement and filled the crown.				
2. Seated the provisional coverage and allowed the cement to set.				
3. Removed any excess cement and checked the occlusion.				
4. Provided the patient with home care instructions.				

Competency 51-4 continued

Criteria	Peer	Self	Instructor	Comment
5. Maintained patient comfort and followed appropriate infection control measures throughout the procedure.				

Total amount of points earned _____

Grade _____   *Instructor's initials* _____

Competency 52-1, 52-2 | Delivery of the Partial and the Complete Denture

Performance Objective: The student will assist as needed throughout the preparation and place-ment of a complete and/or partial denture.

Grading Criteria:

3	Student meets most of the criteria without assistance
2	Student requires assistance to meet the stated criteria
1	Student did not prepare accordingly for the stated criteria
0	Not applicable

Criteria	Peer	Self	Instructor	Comment
Preliminary Visits				
1. Exposed radiographs as requested.				
2. Prepared diagnostic casts as requested.				
3. If necessary, prepared a custom tray.				
Preparation Visit				
1. Assisted the dentist during preparation of the teeth.				
2. Assisted in obtaining the final impression, opposing arch impression, and intraoral occlusal registration.				
3. Disinfected the completed impressions.				
4. Recorded the shade and type of artificial teeth on the patient's chart.				
5. Prepared the case for shipment to the commercial laboratory.				
Try-In Visit(s)				
1. Before the patient's appointment, determined that the case had been returned from the laboratory.				
2. Assisted the dentist during try-in and adjustment of the appliance.				

Competency 52-1, 52-2 *continued*

Criteria	Peer	Self	Instructor	Comment
3. When the appliance was removed, disinfected it and prepared the case to be returned to the laboratory for completion.				
Delivery Visit				
1. Before the patient's appointment, determined that the completed case had been returned from the laboratory.				
2. Assembled the appropriate setup.				
3. Assisted the dentist in making any necessary adjustments.				
4. Provided the patient with home care instructions.				

Total amount of points earned _____

Grade _____   *Instructor's initials* _____

| Competency 54-1 | Perform an Electric Pulp Vitality Test |

Performance Objective: In states where it is legal, the student will accurately perform an electric pulp vitality test.

Grading Criteria:

__3__	Student meets most of the criteria without assistance
__2__	Student requires assistance to meet the stated criteria
__1__	Student did not prepare accordingly for the stated criteria
__0__	Not applicable

Note: See chapter to review for this competency.

Criteria	Peer	Self	Instructor	Comment
1. Gathered the appropriate setup.				
2. Described the procedure to the patient.				
3. Identified the tooth to be tested and an appropriate control tooth.				
4. Isolated the teeth to be tested and dried them thoroughly.				
5. Set the control dial at zero.				
6. Placed a thin layer of toothpaste on the tip of the pulp tester electrode.				
7. Tested the control tooth first. Placed the tip of the electrode on the facial surface of the tooth at the cervical third.				
8. Gradually increased the level of the current until the patient felt a response. Recorded the response on the patient's chart.				
9. Repeated the procedure on the suspected tooth and recorded the response on the patient's chart.				

Competency 54-1 continued

Criteria	Peer	Self	Instructor	Comment
10. Maintained patient comfort and followed appropriate infection control measures throughout the procedure.				

Total amount of points earned _____

Grade _____   *Instructor's initials* _____

| Competency 54-2 | Assist in Root Canal Therapy |

Performance Objective: The student will make pretreatment preparations and assist the dentist throughout the procedure. In states where endodontic expanded functions are permitted, the student will perform those steps.

Grading Criteria:

    __3__ Student meets most of the criteria without assistance

    __2__ Student requires assistance to meet the stated criteria

    __1__ Student did not prepare accordingly for the stated criteria

    __0__ Not applicable

Criteria	Peer	Self	Instructor	Comment
1. Prepared the appropriate setup.				
2. Assisted with the administration of a local anesthetic and the placing and disinfecting of the dental dam.				
3. Anticipated the dentist's needs and assisted throughout the procedure by maintaining moisture control and a clear operating field and by exchanging instruments as necessary.				
4. On request, irrigated the canals gently with a solution of sodium hypochlorite and used the HVE tip to remove the excess solution.				
5. On request, placed a rubber stop at the desired working length for that canal.				
6. Assisted in preparation of the trial-point radiograph.				
7. Exposed and processed the trial-point radiograph.				
8. At a signal from the endodontist, prepared the endodontic sealer.				
9. Dipped a file or Lentulo spiral into the cement and transferred it to the endodontist.				

Competency 54-2 continued

Criteria	Peer	Self	Instructor	Comment
10. Dipped the tip of the gutta-percha point into the sealer and transferred it to the endodontist.				
11. Transferred hand instruments and additional gutta-percha points to the endodontist.				
12. Continued the instrument exchange until the procedure was complete and the tooth was sealed with temporary cement.				
13. Exposed and processed a post-treatment radiograph.				
14. Gave the patient post-treatment instructions.				
15. Maintained patient comfort and followed appropriate infection control measures throughout the procedure.				

Total amount of points earned _____

Grade _____ *Instructor's initials* _____

Competency 55-1

Assisting With a Dental Prophylaxis

Performance Objective: The student will demonstrate the ability to assist with a dental prophy-laxis.

Grading Criteria:

__3__	Student meets most of the criteria without assistance
__2__	Student requires assistance to meet the stated criteria
__1__	Student did not prepare accordingly for the stated criteria
__0__	Not applicable

Note: The operator in this procedure can be the dentist or dental hygienist.

Criteria	Peer	Self	Instructor	Comment
1. Adjusted the light as necessary and was prepared to dry teeth with air when requested to do so.				
2. Provided retraction of the lips, tongue, and cheeks.				
3. Rinsed and evacuated fluid from the patient's mouth.				
4. Exchanged instruments with the operator.				
5. Passed the dental floss and/or tape.				
6. Reinforced oral hygiene instructions when requested to do so.				
7. Maintained patient comfort and followed appropriate infection control measures throughout the procedure.				

Total amount of points earned _____

Grade _____ *Instructor's initials* _____

Competency
55-2

Assisting With a
Gingivectomy/Gingivoplasty

Performance Objective: The student will demonstrate the ability to assist with a gingivectomy and gingivoplasty procedure.

Grading Criteria:

__3__	Student meets most of the criteria without assistance
__2__	Student requires assistance to meet the stated criteria
__1__	Student did not prepare accordingly for the stated criteria
__0__	Not applicable

Criteria	Peer	Self	Instructor	Comment
1. Set out patient's health history, radiographs, and periodontal chart.				
2. Anticipated the operator's needs and was prepared to pass and retrieve surgical instruments.				
3. Had gauze ready to remove tissue from instruments.				
4. Provided oral evacuation and retraction.				
5. Irrigated with sterile saline.				
6. Assisted with suture placement.				
7. Placed, or assisted with placement of, the periodontal dressing.				
8. Provided postoperative instructions.				
9. Maintained patient comfort and followed appropriate infection control measures throughout the procedure.				

Total amount of points earned _____

Grade _____   *Instructor's initials* _____

Competency
55-3

Prepare and Place Non-Eugenol
Periodontal Dressing

Performance Objective: The student will demonstrate the ability to prepare and place a non-eugenol periodontal dressing.

Grading Criteria:

___3___ Student meets most of the criteria without assistance

___2___ Student requires assistance to meet the stated criteria

___1___ Student did not prepare accordingly for the stated criteria

___0___ Not applicable

Note: In states where it is legal, the student may place the dressing on a typodont or on a classmate.

Criteria	Peer	Self	Instructor	Comment
Mixing				
1. Extruded equal lengths of the two pastes on a paper pad.				
2. Mixed the pastes until a uniform color was obtained (2–3 minutes).				
3. Placed the material in the paper cup.				
4. Lubricated gloved fingers with saline solution.				
5. Rolled the paste into strips.				
Placement				
1. Pressed small triangle-shaped pieces of dressing into the interproximal spaces.				
2. Adapted one end of the strip around the distal surface of the last tooth in the surgical site.				
3. Gently pressed the remainder of the strip along the incised gingival margin.				
4. Gently pressed the strip into the interproximal areas.				
5. Applied the second strip from the lingual surface.				
6. Joined the facial and lingual strips.				

Competency 55-3 continued

Criteria	Peer	Self	Instructor	Comment
7. Applied gentle pressure on the facial and lingual surfaces.				
8. Checked the dressing for overextension and interference.				
9. Removed any excess dressing, and adjusted the new margins.				
10. Maintained patient comfort and followed appropriate infection control measures throughout the procedure.				

Total amount of points earned _____

Grade _____   *Instructor's initials* _____

Competency 55-4

Removal of Periodontal Dressing

Performance Objective: The student will demonstrate the ability to remove periodontal dressings.

Grading Criteria:

   3   Student meets most of the criteria without assistance

   2   Student requires assistance to meet the stated criteria

   1   Student did not prepare accordingly for the stated criteria

   0   Not applicable

Criteria	Peer	Self	Instructor	Comment
1. Gently inserted the spoon excavator under the margin.				
2. Used lateral pressure to gently pry the dressing away from the tissue.				
3. Checked for sutures and removed any present.				
4. Gently used dental floss to remove all fragments of dressing material.				
5. Irrigated the entire area gently with warm saline solution.				
6. Used the HVE tip or saliva ejector to remove the fluid from the patient's mouth.				
7. Maintained patient comfort and followed appropriate infection control measures throughout the procedure.				

Total amount of points earned _____

Grade _____ *Instructor's initials* _____

Competency 56-2	Performing a Surgical Scrub

Performance Objective: Provided with the appropriate equipment, the student will perform a surgical scrub for a sterile surgical procedure.

Grading Criteria:

__3__	Student meets most of the criteria without assistance
__2__	Student requires assistance to meet the stated criteria
__1__	Student did not prepare accordingly for the stated criteria
__0__	Not applicable

Criteria	Peer	Self	Instructor	Comment
1. Wet hands and forearms with warm water.				
2. Placed antimicrobial soap into hands.				
3. Used a surgical scrub brush to scrub hands and forearms for 8 minutes.				
4. Rinsed hands and forearms thoroughly with warm water.				
5. Accomplished additional washing in 3 minutes without a brush.				
6. Dried hands using a sterile, disposable towel.				

Total amount of points earned _____

Grade _____   *Instructor's initials* _____

Competency 56-4

Assisting in a Forceps Extraction

Performance Objective: Provided with information concerning the type of surgery, the tooth, and the type of anesthetics used, the student will prepare the setup, prepare the patient, and assist in a surgical procedure.

Grading Criteria:

　　3　　Student meets most of the criteria without assistance

　　2　　Student requires assistance to meet the stated criteria

　　1　　Student did not prepare accordingly for the stated criteria

　　0　　Not applicable

Criteria	Peer	Self	Instructor	Comment
Treatment Room Preparation				
1. Prepared the treatment room.				
2. Kept instruments in their sterile wraps until ready for use. If a surgical tray was preset, opened the tray and placed a sterile towel over the instruments.				
3. Placed the appropriate local anesthetic on the tray.				
4. Placed the appropriate forceps on the tray.				
Patient Preparation				
1. Seated the patient, and placed a sterile patient drape or towel.				
2. Took patient's vital signs and recorded them in the patient's record.				
3. Adjusted the dental chair to the proper position.				
4. Stayed with the patient until the dentist entered the treatment room.				
During the Surgical Procedure				
1. Maintained the chain of asepsis.				
2. Monitored vital signs.				

Competency 56-4 continued

Criteria	Peer	Self	Instructor	Comment
3. Aspirated and retracted as needed.				
4. Transferred and received instruments as needed.				
5. Maintained a clear operating field with adequate light and irrigation.				
6. Steadied the patient's head and mandible if necessary.				
7. Observed the patient's condition and anticipated the dentist's needs.				
8. Maintained patient comfort and followed appropriate infection control measures throughout the procedure.				

Total amount of points earned _____

Grade _____ *Instructor's initials* _____

Competency 56-8 | Suture Removal

Performance Objective: Given the appropriate setup, the student will remove sutures.

Grading Criteria:

__3__	Student meets most of the criteria without assistance
__2__	Student requires assistance to meet the stated criteria
__1__	Student did not prepare accordingly for the stated criteria
__0__	Not applicable

Note: In some states, this procedure is legal for the dental assistant to perform.

Criteria	Peer	Self	Instructor	Comment
1. The dentist examined the surgical site and instructed the assistant to remove the sutures.				
2. Wiped the area with an antiseptic agent.				
3. Held the suture away from the tissue with cotton pliers.				
4. Cut the suture with suture scissors, making sure the scissors were lying flat near the tissue.				
5. Grasped the knot with cotton pliers and removed it, keeping away from the tissue.				
6. Counted the number of sutures removed and recorded it in the patient's chart.				
7. Maintained patient comfort and followed appropriate infection control measures throughout the procedure.				

Total amount of points earned _____

Grade _____   *Instructor's initials* _____

Competency 57-2	Assist in the Placement of a Stainless Steel Crown

Performance Objective: The student will assist in the preparation and placement of a stainless steel crown.

Grading Criteria:

    3   Student meets most of the criteria without assistance

    2   Student requires assistance to meet the stated criteria

    1   Student did not prepare accordingly for the stated criteria

    0   Not applicable

Criteria	Peer	Self	Instructor	Comment
1. Gathered the appropriate setup.				
2. Assisted in the administration of the local anesthetic.				
3. Assisted in the sizing of the stainless steel crown.				
4. Transferred instruments as requested in the transfer zone.				
5. Assisted in the trimming and contouring of the stainless steel crown.				
6. Prepared cement and assisted in the cementation of the stainless steel crown.				
7. Maintained patient comfort and followed appropriate infection control measures throughout the procedure.				

Total amount of points earned _____

Grade _____ *Instructor's initials* _____

Competency 57-3 | Assist in the Reimplantment of an Avulsed Tooth

Performance Objective: The student will assist in the reimplantment of an avulsed tooth.

Grading Criteria:

　　3　Student meets most of the criteria without assistance

　　2　Student requires assistance to meet the stated criteria

　　1　Student did not prepare accordingly for the stated criteria

　　0　Not applicable

Note: See chapter to review for this competency.

Criteria	Peer	Self	Instructor	Comment
1. Gathered the appropriate setup.				
2. Assisted in the administration of the local anesthetic.				
3. Assisted as needed throughout the procedure.				
4. Exposed the postoperative radiograph.				
5. Maintained patient comfort and followed appropriate infection control measures throughout the procedure.				

Total amount of points earned _____

Grade _____ *Instructor's initials* _____

Competency 58-1	Rubber Cup Coronal Polishing

Performance Objective: In states where coronal polishing by a dental assistant is legal, the student will perform a complete mouth coronal polish.

Grading Criteria:

    __3__ Student meets most of the criteria without assistance

    __2__ Student requires assistance to meet the stated criteria

    __1__ Student did not prepare accordingly for the stated criteria

    __0__ Not applicable

Criteria	Peer	Self	Instructor	Comment
1. Gathered appropriate supplies.				
2. Prepared the patient and explained the procedure.				
3. Maintained the correct operator position and posture for each quadrant.				
4. Maintained adequate retraction and an appropriate fulcrum for each quadrant.				
5. Used the rubber polishing cup and abrasive with the proper polishing movements in all quadrants.				
6. Used the bristle brush and abrasive properly in all quadrants.				
7. Controlled handpiece speed and pressure throughout while maintaining patient safety and comfort.				
8. Flossed between the patient's teeth.				
9. Rinsed the patient's mouth.				
10. Evaluated the coronal polish. Repeated parts as necessary.				

Competency 58-1 continued

Criteria	Peer	Self	Instructor	Comment
11. Maintained patient comfort and followed appropriate infection control measures throughout the procedure.				

Total amount of points earned _____

Grade _____   *Instructor's initials* _____

Competency 59-1	Application of Dental Sealants

Performance Objective: In states where it is legal for the dental assistant to do so, the student will apply pit and fissure sealants.

Grading Criteria:
- 3 — Student meets most of the criteria without assistance
- 2 — Student requires assistance to meet the stated criteria
- 1 — Student did not prepare accordingly for the stated criteria
- 0 — Not applicable

Criteria	Peer	Self	Instructor	Comment
1. Gathered appropriate supplies.				
2. Seated the patient and explained the procedure.				
3. Polished the teeth to be treated.				
4. Used appropriate steps to prevent contamination by moisture or saliva.				
5. Placed the etching agent on the appropriate surfaces for the time specified by the manufacturer.				
6. Rinsed and dried the teeth and then verified the appearance of the etched surfaces. If the appearance was not satisfactory, etched the surfaces again.				
7. Placed the sealant on the etched surfaces.				
8. Light-cured the material according to the manufacturer's directions.				
9. Checked the occlusion and made adjustments as necessary.				
10. Asked the dentist (instructor) to evaluate the procedure before the patient was dismissed.				

Competency 59-1 continued

Criteria	Peer	Self	Instructor	Comment
11. Maintained patient comfort and followed appropriate infection control measures throughout the procedure.				

Total amount of points earned _____

Grade _____   *Instructor's initials* _____

Competency
60-1 through 60-3 | Placement of Separators

Performance Objective: The student will demonstrate the ability to place separators.

Grading Criteria:

__3__	Student meets most of the criteria without assistance
__2__	Student requires assistance to meet the stated criteria
__1__	Student did not prepare accordingly for the stated criteria
__0__	Not applicable

Criteria	Peer	Self	Instructor	Comment
1. Gathered the appropriate setup.				
2. Explained the procedure to the patient.				
3. Carried the separator with the appropriate instrument for placement.				
4. Inserted the separator below the proximal contact.				
5. Correct amount of separators placed.				
6. Provided postoperative instructions to the patient.				
7. Maintained patient comfort throughout the procedure and followed appropriate infection control measures throughout the procedure.				

Total amount of points earned _____

Grade _____ *Instructor's initials* _____

Competency 60-4	Assist in the Fitting and Cementation of Orthodontic Bands

Performance Objective: The student will prepare the appropriate setup and assist in the cementation of orthodontic bands.

Grading Criteria:

__3__	Student meets most of the criteria without assistance
__2__	Student requires assistance to meet the stated criteria
__1__	Student did not prepare accordingly for the stated criteria
__0__	Not applicable

Criteria	Peer	Self	Instructor	Comment
1. Gathered the appropriate setup.				
2. Placed each preselected orthodontic band on a small square of masking tape with the occlusal surface on the tape.				
3. Wiped any buccal tubes or attachments with lip balm.				
4. Mixed the cement according to the manufacturer's directions.				
5. Loaded the bands with cement correctly by flowing cement into the band.				
6. Transferred the band correctly.				
7. For a maxillary band, transferred the band pusher.				
8. For a mandibular band, transferred the band seater.				
9. Repeated the process until all of the bands were seated.				
10. Cleaned the cement spatula and slab.				
11. Used a scaler or explorer to remove the excess cement on the enamel surfaces, then rinsed the patient's mouth.				

Competency 60-4 continued

Criteria	Peer	Self	Instructor	Comment
12. Maintained patient comfort throughout the procedure and followed appropriate infection control measures throughout the procedure.				

Total amount of points earned _____

Grade _____   *Instructor's initials* _____

Competency 60-5

Assist in the Direct Bonding of Orthodontic Brackets

Performance Objective: The student will prepare the appropriate setup and assist in the bonding of orthodontic brackets.

Grading Criteria:

    __3__ Student meets most of the criteria without assistance

    __2__ Student requires assistance to meet the stated criteria

    __1__ Student did not prepare accordingly for the stated criteria

    __0__ Not applicable

Criteria	Peer	Self	Instructor	Comment
1. Gathered the appropriate setup.				
2. If stain or plaque was present, the tooth surfaces were prepared using rubber cup and pumice slurry.				
3. Isolated the teeth.				
4. Assisted throughout the etching of the teeth.				
5. Applied a small quantity of bonding material on the back of the bracket.				
6. Used bracket placement tweezers to transfer the bracket to the orthodontist.				
7. Transferred an orthodontic scaler for final placement and the removal of excess bonding material.				
8. Repeated steps 5, 6, and 7 until all brackets were bonded.				

Competency 60–5 continued

Criteria	Peer	Self	Instructor	Comment
9. Maintained patient comfort and followed appropriate infection control measures throughout the procedure.				

Total amount of points earned _____

Grade _____ *Instructor's initials* _____

Competency
60-7

Place and Remove Ligature Ties

Performance Objective: The student will place and remove wire ligatures and elastomeric ligature ties.

Grading Criteria:

    3   Student meets most of the criteria without assistance

    2   Student requires assistance to meet the stated criteria

    1   Student did not prepare accordingly for the stated criteria

    0   Not applicable

Criteria	Peer	Self	Instructor	Comment
Wire Ligature Placement				
1. Gathered the appropriate setup.				
2. Placed the ligature around the bracket, and used the ligature director to push the wire against the tie wing.				
3. Properly twisted the ends of the ligature together.				
4. Used the hemostat to twist the wire snugly against the bracket. Repeated the procedure until all brackets were ligated.				
5. Used a ligature cutter to cut the excess wire, leaving a 4- to 5-mm pigtail.				
6. Tucked the pigtails under the arch wire using the correct instruments.				
7. Determined that nothing was protruding that might injure the patient.				
Wire Ligature Removal				
1. Held the ligature cutter properly and used the beaks of the pliers to cut the wire at easiest access.				
2. Carefully unwrapped the ligature and removed it.				

Competency 60-7 continued

Criteria	Peer	Self	Instructor	Comment
3. Did not twist or pull as the ligatures were cut and removed.				
4. Continued cutting and removing until all brackets were untied.				
5. Maintained patient comfort and followed appropriate infection control measures throughout the procedure.				

Elastomeric Tie Placement

1. Gathered the appropriate setup.				
2. Used a hemostat and placed the beaks of the pliers on a tie, then closed the pliers.				
3. Placed the tie on the gingival portion of one tie wing and slipped the tie around the edges of the bracket.				
4. Released the pliers.				

Elastomeric Tie Removal

1. Used the orthodontic scaler held in a pen grasp and supported the teeth and tissue with the other hand.				
2. Placed the scaler tip between the bracket tie wings, and pulled the tie at the gingival position with a rolling motion.				
3. Removed the tie in an occlusal direction.				

Competency 60-7 continued

Criteria	Peer	Self	Instructor	Comment
4. Maintained patient comfort and followed appropriate infection control measures throughout the procedure.				

Total amount of points earned _____

Grade _____   *Instructor's initials* _____

Competency 64-1	Preparing a Professional Résumé

Performance Objective: Given a computer, printer, and paper, the student will prepare a one-page résumé.

Grading Criteria:

3	Student meets most of the criteria without assistance
2	Student requires assistance to meet the stated criteria
1	Student did not prepare accordingly for the stated criteria
0	Not applicable

Criteria	Peer	Self	Instructor	Comment
1. The résumé was one page in length.				
2. Used white or ivory bond paper.				
3. Used common typefaces.				
4. Used a 10-, 12-, or 14-point font size.				
5. Used 1-inch margins on all sides.				
6. Résumé was neat and error free.				
7. Résumé was concise and easy to read.				

Total amount of points earned _____

Grade _____ *Instructor's initials* _____